YOUR COMPLETE GUIDE TO

Breast Reduction

& Breast Lifts

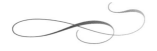

Alain Polynice, M.D.
Aloysius Smith, M.D.

Addicus Books
Omaha, Nebraska

An Addicus Nonfiction Book

Copyright 2006 by Alain Polynice, M.D., and Aloysius Smith, M.D.
All rights reserved. No part of this publication may be reproduced, stored in a retrieval system, or transmitted in any form or by any means, electronic, mechanical, photocopied, recorded, or otherwise, without the prior written permission of the publisher. For information, write Addicus Books, Inc., P.O. Box 45327, Omaha, Nebraska 68145.

ISBN# 1-886039-17-8

Cover design by Peri Poloni-Gabriel, www.knockoutbooks.com
Interior design by Melissa Marquardt, www.abacusgraphics.com
Illustrations by Jack Kusler

This book is not intended to serve as a substitute for a physician.
Nor is it the authors' intent to give medical advice contrary to that of an attending physician.

Library of Congress Cataloging-in-Publication Data

Polynice, Alain, 1965-
  Your complete guide to breast reduction and breast lifts / Alain Polynice, Aloysius Smith.
    p. cm.
  Includes index.
  ISBN 1-886039-17-8 (alk. paper)
  1. Reduction mammaplasty—Popular works. 2. Breast—Surgery—Popular works. 3. Surgery, Plastic—Popular works. I. Smith, Aloysius, 1949- II. Title.

RD539.8.P64 2006
618.1'90592—dc22

2005031976

Addicus Books, Inc.
Addicus Books
P.O. Box 45327
Omaha, NE 68145
Web site: www.AddicusBooks.com

Printed in the United States of America
10 9 8 7 6 5 4 3 2 1

Contents

Introduction...vi

Acknowledgments...vi

1 Contemplating Breast Reduction Surgery 1

2 Choosing a Plastic Surgeon.....................................11

3 Your Consultation..19

4 Preparing for Breast Reduction Surgery....................29

5 Your Surgical Procedure 39

6 Breast Lifts..57

7 Follow-up Care 71

8 The New You! 79

Resources 85

Glossary 88

Index 94

About the Authors..99

Introduction

If you are interested in breast reduction, you are like millions of women who are concerned about the appearance of their breasts. Whether the changes are due to aging, weight gain, weight loss, or childbirth, large breasts can be burdensome, both physically and emotionally.

Breast reductions and breast lifts can be the most challenging procedures in plastic surgery. No two breasts are alike, and achieving symmetry while keeping the scars at a minimum can be difficult. They can also be the most rewarding operations for both the patient and the surgeon. Often breasts cause significant physical pain and discomfort due to sheer size and weight, but even more important are the emotional and psychological effects of women not feeling comfortable in their own bodies. There is no greater reward for the surgeon than having a patient say she has experienced physical relief and now feels more self-confident and more at ease in her own skin.

If you are considering a breast reduction or a breast lift, we hope this book will guide you and provide you with information you need to make the right choice for you.

Acknowledgments

Without the love and support of my family, this book would never have become a reality. To my parents for their unwavering faith and encouragement which showed me that nothing was impossible, and to Allison, my wife and colleague, who never lets me sell myself short and allows me to strive for ever-higher goals.

I also owe an immense debt of gratitude to my teachers and mentors for their guidance and to my students for keeping me on my toes. I would also like to thank Alyson Meadows for her editorial help in putting this book together.

Last, but not least, a special thanks to all my patients, for whom this book was written. My greatest satisfaction is being able to provide you with the latest techniques and also use what I learn from you to further advance the field of breast surgery.

Alain Polynice, M.D.

The techniques used for breast reduction surgery have evolved over many years. We owe a great deal of gratitude to the innovators of the various techniques that have brought us to the to the stage we're at today. I wish to thank my mother for setting no limits on achievement. I also wish to thank Dr. William Stahl for defining leadership by example and Dr. John Woods for believing that plastic surgery training was not only for the selected few. I also thank Dr. P. G. Arnold for his friendship and guidance.

Aloysius Smith, M.D.

Where nature finishes producing its shapes, there man begins,
with natural things and with the help of nature itself,
to create infinite varieties of shapes.

— Leonardo da Vinci

CHAPTER ONE

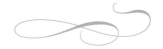

Contemplating Breast Reduction Surgery

1

Contemplating Breast Reduction Surgery

If you have large breasts, you are all too familiar with the frustrations that may come with having them. You know what it feels like to have people "talking to your chest." Perhaps you avoid days at the beach or pool because you feel self-conscious of your large breasts. Have you ever turned down offers from friends to shop for clothes because of the embarrassment you feel when shirts and dresses don't fit across your chest? Do you turn down the invitation to participate in physical activities?

If you answered "yes" to these questions, you're not alone. Many women feel restricted by their bodies and actually avoid certain activities that others enjoy because of this discomfort. They don't remember the last time they felt carefree at the beach. They don't even try on sexy lingerie anymore, because they know it won't fit quite right. All of this is because they are not comfortable with their own breasts.

What might life be like without large, heavy breasts? Maybe you'd notice people paying attention to you and not just your chest. Maybe you'd exercise at the gym without pain. Maybe you'd stand taller, because you wouldn't feel self-conscious about your breasts. There's a good chance that you'd notice a difference in the way you feel, the way you move, and how you carry yourself.

How Breasts Develop

Think back to your adolescent years for a moment, back to when it all began. Some girls developed breasts early and some were late bloomers. Either way, it seemed that very few were pleased with the rate of their development. Some girls, embarrassed, changed for gym class in bathrooms down the hall, instead of the locker rooms to hide the fact that their breasts were more fully developed than many of the other girls'. Other girls, equally ashamed, tried to hide their underdeveloped breasts and wondered when on earth they would ever catch up to the others.

These girls were simply caught in various stages of breast development. Breast growth is one of the earliest indications that puberty has begun. The process begins with the secretion of hormones from the pituitary gland, at the base of the brain. This gland controls bodily functions such as growth and ovary production. It's common for breasts to begin to grow sometime between the ages of eight and twelve. Whenever the onset of breast development, it's likely that breasts will continue to grow for approximately four years after girls begin menstruating.

Breasts develop in five separate stages. The first stage is actually the flat chest that children have before development begins. Stage two begins when children begin to bud, meaning that their breasts form small peaks as nipples swell, and tenderness sets in. The third stage of breast development starts when adolescents begin to build fat in their breast tissue. Breasts grow more rapidly in this stage than in any other. Often, it's during this time that girls begin to menstruate. After this point, breast size does not usually increase much; instead, during stage four, the shape of the breasts changes as the nipples begin to protrude. Only during the teenage years will nipples point straight

Breast Anatomy

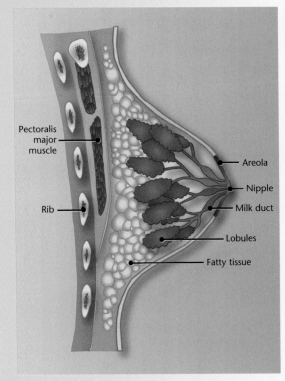

Pectoralis major muscle

Rib

Areola

Nipple

Milk duct

Lobules

Fatty tissue

A woman suffering with large breasts needs to know that she has options. With new techniques in breast reduction with minimal scars we can offer relief from the physical discomfort associated with large breasts and dramatically improve self-image.

— Alain Polynice, M.D.

ahead and not sag at all. Stage five is full maturation, and breast development is complete. This entire process should conclude around age seventeen or eighteen. Permanent breast size should be evident at this point.

Why Some Woman Have Large Breasts

All of us have the same basic breast anatomy, so why does breast size vary so much from woman to woman? The answer is deceptively simple—fat! It's true. We all do have roughly the same number of *breast ducts* and *lobules*, which allow lactation to occur, but we do have different amounts of fat deposited within our breasts.

Genetics

Breast size is generally determined by genetics. In fact, breast size has much more to do with your genes than it does with your hormones or diet. This fact can be confusing, though, if your breast size greatly differs from that of your mother's or your sister's. Understanding genes is sometimes tricky, because they're complex. Your genes are derived not only from your mother's but also from your father's side of the family. You may have a breast size similar to many of your close female relatives, or you may take after your Great-Aunt Betty.

Estrogen

Estrogen is a hormone that surges during puberty, ages eleven to fifteen, and during pregnancy. Any increase in estrogen levels causes breasts to enlarge. Although breasts do become enlarged during pregnancy because of the increase in estrogen, they often shrink and sag after childbirth or after breastfeeding ceases. Usually breasts will regain some of their previous fullness a few months afterward.

The use of oral contraceptives or post-menopause estrogen replacement pills may enhance breast size because of their estrogen content.

Weight Gain

Gaining weight will typically cause the breasts to become bigger. However, breasts usually return to their previous size once weight is lost.

Evolution of Cosmetic Breast Surgery

It's believed that the first breast reduction surgery was performed by an English doctor, William Durston, in 1669. Since then, a variety of innovative and skilled surgeons have perfected breast reduction techniques that maximize results and minimize risks.

What Is Breast Reduction Surgery?

Breast reduction surgery, also referred to as a *reduction mammoplasty*, is a surgical procedure that involves reducing the size, weight, and mass of the breasts. This is accomplished by excising fat, skin, and glandular tissue. The skin is then pulled together and sutured. As a result of this surgery, the breasts are smaller and more shapely. Although the intent of breast reduction surgery is to decrease the size and weight of the breasts, the procedure also lifts the breasts to correct drooping. This procedure is most commonly performed on women who have large, pendulous breasts, which may be causing both physical problems and social embarrassment.

The number of women seeking breast reduction has remained steady over the past few years. According to the American Society of Plastic Surgeons (ASPS) more than 100,000 women have breast reduction surgery annually.

Reasons for Breast Reduction Surgery

Physical Reasons

Most people seem to think of large breasts as a symbol of beauty and attractiveness. However, many women with large breasts consider them more of a curse than a blessing. They complain of a variety of physical ailments, including neck, back, and shoulder pain, *bra strap grooving,* skeletal deformities, rashes underneath their breasts, trouble breathing, difficulty exercising, and poor posture.

Emotional Reasons

Physical symptoms are not the extent of a woman's plight if she is burdened with large breasts. Often, these women also experience a range of significant emotional issues—from self-consciousness to self-esteem problems—because their breasts have been the topic of teasing and objectification since puberty. Because these women view their chests as unattractive or the source of too much attention, they work hard not to reveal this area to anyone else, especially those whose opinions they value most. This means that they often don't feel comfortable changing their clothes in front of others, which may cause them to avoid sports activities or fitness centers or even sex sometimes. Are you one of these women?

Are You a Candidate for Breast Reduction?

If any of this sounds familiar and you are in good health overall, you may be a candidate for breast reduction surgery. Breast reduction surgery has helped thousands of women—from teenagers to ladies in their eighties—feel more comfortable physically and emotionally. To be a breast surgery candidate, you need to be in good general health. If you do have a medical condition, such as diabetes, you may still be able to have your procedure performed, but you'll need to follow your surgeon's recommendations.

Most plastic surgeons recommend that women wait until they are at least eighteen to twenty years old before they consider undergoing breast surgery of any kind, to make sure that their breast development is complete. The exception to this rule is teenagers who suffer from *virginal breast hypertrophy*—the condition of having developed large breasts at a very early age, usually during grade school. When this condition is present, many surgeons will feel comfortable performing a breast reduction to increase the adolescent's quality of life and decrease any related physical symptoms.

When Breast Reduction Surgery Might Not Be for You

If you are currently pregnant or breastfeeding, you are not a breast surgery candidate right now, in part because of the adverse effects anesthesia could have on your unborn baby. In fact, it's a good idea to delay breast surgery until after your last child breastfeeds because the results of your surgery could be reversed with another pregnancy or period of breastfeeding.

If You Are Overweight

You may not be a candidate for breast surgery if you are obese or overweight. Many surgeons will not perform breast surgery until patients have reached a stable weight because surgery results will not be optimal; further, the results would be lost after a dramatic weight loss—sagging would occur.

Also, your insurance company may refuse to pay for your surgery if it learns you have not tried to lose weight first. A good starting point

My advice to women considering breast surgery. Do the research. Find a good surgeon. Do it. I have no regrets. This surgery changed my life. I have confidence again.

— Liz, 32

may be a weight-loss program consisting of a nutrition plan and an exercise regimen that your doctor recommends. This way, you'll know for sure whether you actually require a breast reduction or if you just needed to loose a few pounds to feel good about your body again.

If You Smoke

If you are a smoker, you are not an ideal candidate for any type of surgery. Nicotine restricts blood flow in smaller blood vessels, and as a result, the blood cannot move oxygen efficiently to help the body heal from surgery. At the very least, a plastic surgeon will recommend you stop smoking for several weeks before and after the procedure. Excessive alcohol consumption, marijuana smoking, and steroid use will also increase your risk of complications during and after surgery.

If You Have Major Health Concerns

Generally speaking, it's not safe to undergo any kind of surgery if you have any major medical condition, but often it can be controlled enough to make breast surgery possible for you. Your surgeon can usually refer you back to your general practitioner, who can often create a plan to prepare you for surgery. You may need to closely follow your doctor's instructions for a designated period of time, though, before he or she will consider surgery safe for you. Once your doctor is confident in your ability to safely have surgery, you will be released for your breast procedure.

If You Develop Keloid Scars

Some individuals are prone to develop keloid scars—fleshy masses of scars. Unfortunately, this condition is very difficult to treat, and those who are aware of their vulnerability to keloids should seriously reconsider undergoing breast surgery. Most people who are at risk for this condition already know it, because they probably have developed keloids at some earlier point in their lives. If you think you are prone to forming keloids, ask your surgeon if he or she has experience with patients who have developed them; a surgeon can take actions which may minimize the formation of severe keloid scars.

Making the Decision

Surgery is serious—it poses risks, discomfort, and a significant recovery period. Breast surgery is not something to take lightly or commit to impulsively.

Despite the inconvenience, many women who have undergone breast reduction surgery report that they would do it all again. They say they have a whole new lease on life once they recover from their procedures, finding themselves able to exercise in ways they never could before and being more active than ever. They continually discover new physical activities they enjoy and often meet new friends in the process. These women also report that their personal lives dramatically improve with their newfound confidence. They state that their lives are much more fulfilling.

CHAPTER TWO

Choosing a Plastic Surgeon

2

Choosing a Plastic Surgeon

*I*f you wish to further explore breast reduction surgery, it's now time to choose a plastic surgeon to perform your procedure. You may already know about the plastic surgeon whom you wish to perform your surgery. If you don't have a surgeon in mind, you'll need to do some searching. Finding a competent plastic surgeon with whom you feel comfortable is essential to achieving your desired results.

It's important to keep two things in mind as you embark on your quest for the ideal plastic surgeon—a surgeon's competence to deliver the results you are looking for and his or her ability to make you feel comfortable throughout the entire process. Thoroughly researching a surgeon's qualifications is key, but don't forget to follow your instincts as you search for the right plastic surgeon for you.

Finding a Plastic Surgeon

You will need to find a surgeon who is experienced in breast surgery. In fact, breast surgery should be a significant part of the surgeon's practice, not just a procedure that he or she performs from time to time. There are several ways to find a plastic surgeon.

Referrals

If you have any friends who have undergone breast surgery, ask them if they are pleased with their results. If they are, inquire about what they appreciated, specifically, about the process. Then ask them who performed their operations.

You may also be able to get referrals from your *general practitioner* or *gynecologist*. These physicians may know several local plastic surgeons, and they may have even seen their work in patients they have in common.

Internet Searches

If you're interested in doing some online research, one of the best Web sites for obtaining overall information about plastic surgery procedures and board-certified plastic surgeons is that of the American Society of Plastic Surgeons (ASPS). Another resource is PlasticSurgery.com, which provides viewers with local plastic surgeon referrals and links to pertinent sites.

Training and Experience of the Plastic Surgeon

For most of us, trying to understand the qualifications and credentials of plastic surgeons is a bit confusing. Here's an overview of the process of training and education. Plastic surgery requires years of specialized training, starting with medical school. To become a plastic surgeon, the surgeon must first have graduated from medical school, and have a license in the state to practice medicine. The medical school should be "accredited," which means that the school meets standards set by a national authority for medical education programs.

Once graduated from medical school, a plastic surgeon must complete a minimum of six to seven years of additional training in a

The key to choosing a plastic surgeon is communication, establishing a good rapport. Then, a patient can then feel comfortable and be confident that her surgeon understands her problem and can lead her in the right direction.

— Alain Polynice, M.D.

hospital where he or she is performing surgery. This is often a combination of general and plastic surgery. This period of training is called a residency. So, by the time a surgeon goes into practice, he or she has had plenty of real, hands-on experience working side by side with senior surgeons.

A plastic surgeon's training is ongoing. Surgeons are required to take continuing medical education courses to keep their certification up-to-date.

Board Certification: What Does It Mean?

Perhaps you have heard that it is important to go to a plastic surgeon who is "board certified." What does this mean? Being board certified means that after the surgeon has completed residency training, he or she has passed a rigorous written exam, which is followed by an oral exam. These tests are given by a recognized board of senior physicians who oversee the plastic surgery specialty. Once the surgeon has passed these tests, board certification is granted. Any plastic surgeon you consider should be certified by the American Board of Surgery as well as the American Board of Plastic Surgery.

Once certified, a surgeon must continually update his or her credentials in order to be recertified. This recertification is usually required every ten years. Throughout this period, the surgeon will have receives additional training annually through continuing education coursework.

Board certification is a completely voluntary process. Surgeons are not required to be certified to perform surgery; however, if you want peace of mind knowing that your plastic surgeon meets important requirements set by an independent board, choose a board-certified one. You can verify a surgeon's certification at the American Board of Surgery Web site at www.abms.org.

Finally, just like any other doctor, your surgeon needs to be licensed to practice medicine in your state. There's nothing voluntary about licensing—it's required. Your surgeon must have a valid, current license issued by the state's medical licensing board in order to legally practice in the state. Licensing criteria differ slightly from one state to another. If you need further information about a surgeon's licensure, you may check with your state's medical board to learn more about licensing and license verification.

Experience of the Plastic Surgeon

Most plastic surgeons you'll talk to will be well trained and certified. But what about their level of experience? You'll want to select a surgeon who has experience with the breast surgery procedures you're considering.

So, how much experience should the surgeon have? We often hear that it's important to ask a surgeon how many procedures like the one you're considering he or she has performed. But it may be difficult for you to know what a "right" answer is. Is it five such procedures a year, or is it fifty? To have an appropriate level of experience, most plastic surgeons would recommend that the surgeon you choose complete at least several surgical procedures, like the one you're planning, several times a month on a regular basis.

Finally, a surgeon who is experienced will know how to select the right patients for cosmetic breast surgery. Not all women are good candidates when they first visit a plastic surgeon, but perhaps they will be later on. An experienced plastic surgeon will know who should and who shouldn't have the surgery.

Make sure you choose a surgeon who has a good bedside manner. Ask a lot of questions so that you feel comfortable going into the procedure.

— Brenda, 33

Additional Methods to Check Surgeon Credibility

Another way to ensure that your prospective plastic surgeon is well qualified is to call your state's medical board or visit its Web site. This information is in the public domain, so you'll be able to access any information about his or her having been disciplined for inappropriate practices. Be aware that a search of your state's records would not provide information about any other state in which a surgeon may have practiced.

If you'd like to carry your research one step further, you could even contact the hospital where the surgeon you're considering practices. The hospital can give you a general sense of the surgeon's performance and reputation.

Rapport with Your Plastic Surgeon

It is important to feel comfortable with the plastic surgeon who will perform your surgery. Once you have met with a plastic surgeon, ask yourself how you felt about the meeting. This is just as essential as diligently asking questions about the surgical procedure you are considering. Before you make your final decision, ask yourself the following questions:

- Is the surgeon someone with whom I feel comfortable?
- Did he or she answer all of my questions about the surgery process?
- Am I confident that I could call my surgeon with any questions that I remember later?
- Does this surgeon respond sensitively to my needs and take my goals seriously?
- Does he or she take enough time to talk with me until I fully

understand the details of my procedure?
- Do I feel safe in the hands of this surgeon?
- Is this surgeon someone whom I trust?

Surgical Center Accreditation

In addition to checking a surgeon's credentials, it's important to assess the safety of the location where he or she performs breast surgery procedures. Some plastic surgeons perform their surgeries in hospitals, in which case you should be in a well-staffed, safely operated environment. Hospitals have a certain level of standards they must meet periodically to continue to provide services to patients. If, however, your surgeon performs breast surgery procedures out of his or her own surgical center, a closer look is warranted.

Surgical centers may or may not have received *accreditation*. Two agencies—the American Association of Accredited Ambulatory Surgical Facilities (AAAASF) and the Accreditation Association for Ambulatory Health Care (AAAHC)—are responsible for inspecting surgical centers and ensuring that they meet the highest standards of safety for patients. This means that all equipment, supplies, and procedures must meet or surpass the high expectations of these two accrediting agencies.

It's not required that surgical centers be accredited; however, those that are accredited operate more safely than those that are not. A surgical center that has been accredited has met the same government requirements regarding safety procedures and sterilization that hospitals must meet. Your surgeon's surgical center should be accredited by at least one of the accrediting organizations.

Questions to Ask the Surgeon

- What are your medical credentials?

- Are you board certified?

- How many breast reduction procedures have you performed?

- Have any complications occurred during or after procedures you've performed?

- May I talk to at least one of your patients who has had this procedure?

- Where will the operation be performed?

- Is your surgery facility accredited?

CHAPTER THREE

Your Consultation

3

Your Consultation

....

*O*nce you have decided on a plastic surgeon, you'll need to schedule a consultation. During your consultation, you'll learn whether you are indeed a likely candidate for breast surgery. If you are, the surgeon you're seeing will explain the details of having cosmetic breast surgery. The consultation is also an opportunity for you to ask questions about the procedure and its probable outcome and risks, as well as those about practical matters, such as cost.

Preparing for Your Consultation

Before you meet with a plastic surgeon, it's important to make sure that you are prepared. Some surgeons may want medical records during the consultation; others may wait until you have actually scheduled a surgery date before they request medical records. Because surgeons have different preferences for when they require medical histories, it's best to call and ask the surgeon's staff what information they'd like for you to take to the consultation.

Either way, you'll need to be prepared to give the surgeon a good overview of your medical history. It's important that your surgeon understand your current physical condition. Be prepared to inform the surgeon of any present or past medical conditions and any surgical procedures you've undergone, too. Also, you'll need to tell the surgeon which prescription drugs you are taking currently and why you are taking them.

What Are Your Goals?

It is essential that you communicate your wishes to the plastic surgeon. You may want to spend some time asking yourself what exactly you want to achieve with cosmetic surgery. What results are you hoping for? Flip through magazines or other photos to help you decide which breast shape, size, and lift are optimal for you. You'll need to have a good idea of what look you want before you speak to your surgeon. Even if you think that your surgery goal is too lofty, tell the surgeon anyway; that way, he or she will understand your intentions. Having an honest dialogue with your surgeon about your expectations is essential. The surgeon can determine whether he or she can achieve the results you seek only if you are thorough in explaining your goals for the breast procedure.

You may wish to visit the library or go online to do some research of your own on breast surgery so you can ask the surgeon educated questions during your consultation. If you do a bit of self-educating, you'll be able to better understand what the surgery involves.

Take a List of Questions

Remember, it is your surgeon's job to answer all of your questions, no matter how foolish or inconsequential you may think they are. Don't be afraid to ask him or her to clarify anything you don't fully understand. This is your body and your money, so this is not the time to just nod and agree if you don't understand. Keep asking until you do.

Consider preparing a list of questions to take with you so you don't forget anything important during your time with your surgeon. What are you confused about, regarding the procedure? If you don't have all of your questions down on paper, you may find yourself bombarded with too much information at once and then think of

Before my breast reduction, my posture was affected. I was often embarrassed about my large breasts. Now, I have more confidence and can move more easily. I can actually jog around a track.

— Joan, 35

several questions later that you wish you had remembered to ask. This will probably happen anyway, to some degree. If you are concerned about feeling too overwhelmed and not being able to remember important details of your consultation, you may want to take a friend with you to take notes as you are speaking to the surgeon. Doing so could help alleviate some confusion later and help you absorb all of the information you've been given.

If you think of additional questions after your initial consultation, you may wish to schedule a second consultation. A second meeting may also help you feel more comfortable committing to the surgical process. Second consultations also offer the opportunity for you to take a trusted friend or family member with you to help you understand and digest any information given to you.

Do You Feel Comfortable?

Not only will you gain valuable information during your consultation, you also will be able to sense whether you and the surgeon have a good rapport. At no point during the consultation should you feel any pressure from the surgeon to participate in surgery.

It's important to choose a surgeon who conveys a sense of caring and concern for patients. The surgeon's attitude and responses during the consultation are clues to your future relationship with him or her, so be attentive. Listen to you instincts. For example, are your questions answered respectfully and thoroughly? Do you innately trust this individual? Does he or she seem impatient or rushed? Is the staff caring and professional? All of these questions need to be answered to your satisfaction before you agree that this surgeon is the one to perform your procedure.

Your Breast Examination

In addition to providing information about your medical history, you will also need to undergo a breast examination. Your surgeon will visually examine your breasts first to make sure no swelling, bulging, or skin malformations exist. The surgeon will also be evaluating several other factors, including bra shoulder strap grooving, current nipple sensitivity, nipple position, and the distance between different parts of your breast. Also, your surgeon will consider your breast size, breast symmetry, chest wall size, shape, height, and weight in order to make appropriate recommendations.

You'll also be asked to lie down on a table for part of the breast exam. At this time, the surgeon will palpate, or touch, your breasts to check for masses or lumps. He or she will use varying amounts of pressure during this procedure to screen for lumps both near the skin's surface and deep within the breast. This part should feel like a massage and should not be uncomfortable.

The surgeon will also gently squeeze your nipple to check for any discharge; blood or pus could be a symptom of infection, mastitis, or breast cancer. The entire procedure is then performed on your other breast. While you are still sitting, your surgeon may feel the lymph nodes in your armpit and around your collarbone; enlarged nodes may be an indication of infection or breast cancer. Your entire breast examination should be painless.

How Much Can Your Breast Size Be Reduced?

The next stage of your consultation consists of your surgeon taking your measurements to help you choose the breast size and shape that is right for your body. You'll work together to determine the amount of breast tissue that needs to be removed. If you're receiving a breast reduction, your new breasts will need to be small enough to alleviate your physical symptoms. It's important not only to pick a size and shape that you like but also to make sure that it is right for you. For your new look to appear natural, you'll need a good fit for your body.

Any amount of reduction is physically possible, but most surgeons will explain that your "new" breasts need to match your height, weight, and body frame in order look natural. Your surgeon will advise you on breast size and shape to meet your individual needs.

Risks, Complications, and Considerations

Some risks, complications, and considerations do exist with breast reduction surgery procedures, just as they do with any type of surgery. Be sure to ask your surgeon about these. He or she should be sensitive to your concerns about the risks of breast surgery and should take them seriously. Hopefully, your surgeon will alleviate most of them by further educating you on the process. Most surgeries go very smoothly, and the risk of serious complications is slim. More details on risks and complications are covered in detail in Chapter 5: Your Surgical Procedure.

Seeing Before-and-After Photographs

Your surgeon will most likely show you before-and-after pictures of former patients who have undergone the procedures that are of interest to you. Usually, he or she will volunteer these photos, but if not, ask to see them. Your surgeon should have many such photographs. If the surgeon can produce only two or three before-and-after shots, it could be a sign that he or she hasn't had a lot of experience doing the procedure under consideration.

Photographs of You

Your surgeon, most likely, also will want to take a "before" picture of your breasts during the consultation. Most surgeons take before-and-after photographs of all of their patients without exception, no matter which procedure the patients are having performed. These photographs then become part of your personal medical record. Your surgeon should show your photographs to you after they are taken, and give you a copy of them if you desire.

The "before" photograph is taken not only to demonstrate the contrast between the old and new you, but also to serve as a guide to help the medical staff plan for your surgery. Pre-operative photographs are used to obtain pre-authorization from insurance companies. The insurance companies don't usually request the "after" pictures; instead, they rely on pathology reports to make any payment determination. The pathology report is based on lab tests conducted on the breast tissue removed.

References from Previous Patients

Your surgeon should also be able to put you in contact with former patients who've had the same surgical procedure done. This way, you have the chance to learn firsthand about having the procedure. Many surgeons do this routinely—they have names of patients who've agreed to speak to new patients.

Don't feel shy about contacting previous patients. Most people who have had your procedure will be excited to share their story with you. Usually, they enjoy telling new patients about how having surgery enhanced their lives. And who better than former patients to give you the candid details of the process? Be sure to inquire about how comfortable the woman felt with the surgeon.

Paying for Your Procedure

The best way to alleviate confusion over the total cost of your surgery is to talk with your surgeon or a designated staff person about

I chose to be very open about telling people I'd had breast reduction. I am so pleased with the results that I show a lot of people my before/after photos.

— Marie, 28

it. Your consultation is a good opportunity to do this. Once you've discussed your breast surgery options with your surgeon and have chosen which procedure you want, it's time for this conversation. In addition to determining the fee for your procedure, you will need to know what additional fees you will be responsible for. All surgeons' protocols are different, but it's fairly common for patients to cover additional costs, such as those for anesthesia, lab tests, pathology tests, compression vests, or prescription drugs.

Insurance

The effects of breast reduction surgery are cosmetic; however, the procedure itself is considered reconstructive surgery, meaning it is considered a "medical necessity." As a result, health insurance companies often pay for the surgery if it is shown that a patient is suffering from a variety of physical symptoms related to large breasts. You'll need to be able to prove that you need to have your breasts reduced to alleviate physical symptoms.

Insurance companies use a variety of criteria to determine whether breast reduction surgery is a medical necessity. Some companies will pay based only on the amount of breast tissue to be removed; this usually means removal of at least 500 grams of tissue, slightly more than one pound from each breast (454 grams equal 1 pound). Other companies use complex formulas to compare the size of the breasts with the overall size of the body. Some companies also consider body mass index (BMI), which assesses one's percentage of body fat, based on the ratio between one's height and weight. And if you are overweight, your insurance company may require you to first lose weight.

Your surgeon can likely tell you whether your procedure would be covered by insurance. It may even be a good idea to call your insurance company before you arrive for your consultation so that you'll know whether you'll need to explore other payment alternatives.

Self-Pay

If insurance does not cover your desired procedure or if you have no insurance at all, you will need to consider self-pay options. The total cost of your breast surgery will depend on the procedure performed and method used, your geographical location, and your individual surgeon.

Other Payment Arrangements

If insurance is not an option for you, your surgeon may advise you on other payment arrangements. Many patients take out their own bank loans through lenders who work closely with their surgeons. Your surgeon should be able to make this kind of referral. Most surgeons will accept credit cards as a means of payment. Some surgeons may agree to accept monthly payments directly from you. However, most surgeons prefer that the total cost of surgery be paid in full before they complete your procedure.

Informed Consent

At some point prior to your surgery, you will be asked to sign an informed consent form. Informed consent is the process by which a patient can participate in choices about her health care. The intent is to ensure that the patient fully understands her health care decisions. This should include understanding the nature of the surgery, alternatives to the procedure, and the risks and benefits of the surgery. Part of informed consent also includes a patient's acceptance for the use of intervention, if needed, to handle complications that could arise.

Questions to Ask during Your Consultation:

- Are my surgery goals realistic?

- What procedure or procedures do you recommend for me?

- What risks, complications, and side effects could I experience?

- How long will the operation take?

- What kind of anesthetic will be used?

- Will I have post-surgical pain?

- Is it likely that my insurance will pay for my procedure? If not, what other payment options do you recommend?

- When can my procedure be performed?

- How soon can I return to work?

CHAPTER FOUR

Preparing for Breast Reduction Surgery

4

Preparing for Breast Reduction Surgery

*O*nce your surgeon has recommended cosmetic breast surgery for you, there are some preparations you'll need to make before the surgery. Preparation requirements and recommendations will vary from surgeon to surgeon, but familiarity with common guidelines can give you some idea of what to expect during the surgery process. Of course, you will need to rely on your own surgeon to give you specific instructions.

Lab Tests You May Need

If you are younger and healthy, you may not be required to undergo any lab tests. On the other hand, your plastic surgeon may require that you have a full physical examination in order to receive pre-operative medical clearance for surgery. This practice may vary among surgeons, but if you are older—say over forty—your surgeon will ask that you have lab tests. Similarly, if your medical history includes conditions such as diabetes or thyroid problems, the surgeon will require lab tests. If these tests are requested, the plastic surgeon will refer you to your family physician or referring doctor for testing.

Pregnancy Test

Regardless of your age, you will need to demonstrate that you are not pregnant; undergoing surgery while pregnant could be harmful to your fetus. You may opt for a *blood pregnancy test* or a *urine pregnancy test*. Often, a surgeon will request a blood pregnancy test during your consultation and an additional urine pregnancy test on the day of surgery.

Mammogram

If you are over age forty, you'll likely be asked to have a *mammogram*. A mammogram is a low-powered X-ray used to examine the entire inner structure of the breast. It's used to screen for a variety of breast maladies, the most common of which is breast cancer. If your surgeon does recommend a mammogram for you, he or she will refer you to a *radiologist* who is specially trained in mammography.

A radiology technologist will most likely perform your actual screening. During your mammogram, each breast will be inserted into the mammogram machine so that pictures may be taken from more than one angle. This will ensure that your breasts are thoroughly assessed for potential problems. After the mammogram, the radiologist will review your results. He or she may share them with you immediately or send them to your referring surgeon.

Complete Blood Count (CBC)

The *complete blood count (CBC)* and blood chemistry tests both require blood to be drawn from a vein in either your arm or your hand. The CBC is a screening and diagnostic test for a variety of diseases. It will also tell the surgeon whether you are anemic; anemia means that you have too few red blood cells. Symptoms of anemia

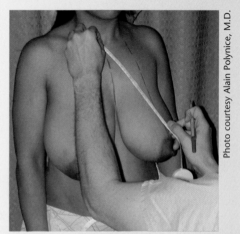

Photo courtesy Alain Polynice, M.D.

Preparing to do breast reduction surgery, the surgeon measures and marks this woman's breasts. The markings serve as a guide for incision placement.

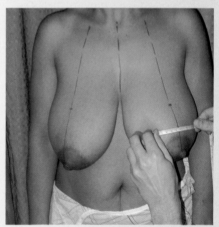

The surgeon measures the areola prior to breast reduction surgery. The size of the areola will also be reduced during the surgery.

include feeling tired, weak, and short of breath. Anyone who is anemic would not be a good candidate for the stress of surgery.

The CBC also indicates whether problems exist with such things as fluid volume, loss of blood, abnormal blood cells, infection, allergies, and clotting ability. The *blood chemistry test* screens for problems with levels of potassium, sodium, creatinine, fasting glucose.

Electrocardiogram (EKG or ECG)

You may be asked to have an *electrocardiogram*, most commonly called an *EKG* or an *ECG*. The purpose of the ECG is to record the electrical activity of your heart and screen for heart disease. This is a painless procedure in which electrodes are affixed to your chest, arms, and legs. It may also include a stress test, in which you may be expected to perform some sort of physical activity, such as walking or running on a treadmill.

Chest X-ray

Your surgeon may request a chest X-ray, as well. The purpose of a chest X-ray is to screen for any lung masses or abnormalities as well as to look at the heart.

Other Preparations for Surgery

Quit Smoking

Whatever your age, one consideration is non-negotiable when it comes to preparing for your surgery: You must quit smoking! Nicotine causes problems with circulation; so, as you can imagine, healing from surgery will pose a problem if you have nicotine in your system. As mentioned earlier, if you smoke, you must stop before and after your surgery. You will need to quit smoking two to three weeks before your surgery and should not smoke until at least two three weeks after surgery. Remember, you won't be able to rely on any of the popular smoking cessation aids that contain nicotine—no nicotine gum, lozenges, or patches. Talk with your surgeon about the best method of quitting for you.

Medication and Diet Restrictions

You'll need to avoid all products containing aspirin for two weeks prior to your surgery date and for one week afterward. Aspirin thins blood and could cause you to bleed excessively during surgery. To decrease the risk of bleeding complications during surgery, you also need to avoid vitamin E, fish oil, and omega-3 supplements for the same reason. After surgery, you will be able to take pain relievers that do not contain aspirin.

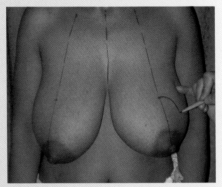
The surgeon continues his markings, guiding him in making incisions along the upper portion of the breast.

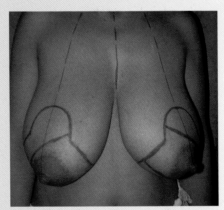
The surgeon has completed markings for an anchor-shaped incision. This technique is often used for removing larger amounts of skin and tissue.

Drugs which May Cause Blood Thinning			
Advil	aspirin	Doan's Pills (Regular & Extra-Strength)	Indocin
Aleve	BC Powder		indomethicin
Alka-Seltzer	BC Cold Powder	Dolobid	Norgesic
Anacin	Bufferin	Dristan	Norgesic Forte
Anaprox	Clinoril	Feldene	Pepto-Bismol (tabs & liquid)
Ansaid	Coricidin	Fiorinal	
Ascriptin	Coumadin	Goody's Headache Powders & Tabs	Percodan
Aspergum	Darvon		Persantine
Aspercream	Darvon with ASA	ibuprofen	
	Disalcid Tabs & Caps		

Before surgery, I squeezed into 36DD bra. My bra straps dug into my shoulders. My back hurt. I had rashes. After surgery, I was a 36C. I am much happier now.

— Mildred, 37

Make sure you speak with your surgeon and receive a complete list of blood-thinning drugs to avoid during your surgery preparation weeks. If in doubt, do not take a drug during this time period without clearing it with your surgeon first. Even "just one" of the wrong medication can make a difference.

Avoid Alcoholic Beverages

Alcohol also thins the blood. Be sure to quit drinking alcohol a few weeks in advance to decrease your risk of related complications during surgery. And, of course, you'll want to make sure that you are eating as healthfully as possible to best prepare your body for surgery.

Arranging for Care after Surgery

Prior to your procedure, you will need to arrange for a reliable friend or relative to transport you home from the hospital or surgical center a couple of hours after your surgery. You will still be experiencing some of the effects of your anesthesia and will not be able to drive yourself home.

Also, you will need care for twenty-four to forty-eight hours after your homecoming. Ask someone with whom you feel comfortable to stay with you during this time to help you with basic tasks. Be aware that if you have young children, you will not be able to care for them for a while, so you will need to make other arrangements for them, as well. You will not be able to care for them or carry them for at least one week, because you'll need time to heal. (If you do care for them too soon, you run the risk of being accidentally hit in the chest by them.) A high level of physical activity early on could be painful and even cause bleeding to occur.

Preparing for Your Return Home

Think ahead to what you will need available to you immediately after your surgery. Prepare to have several items on hand when you come home, especially a variety of fluids, crackers, and your medications filled in advance. Immediately after your procedure, your surgeon most likely will recommend that you restrict your diet to liquids and slowly advance to solid food, since some people do experience nausea after anesthesia. All items you will need after surgery should be located as conveniently as possible. This way, when you arrive home after your procedure, you can actually relax!

The Day before Your Procedure

On the day before your surgery, you'll need to be mindful of a few important details. First of all, this is not the day to run that marathon you've been training for during the past eight months. Vigorous exercise is not recommended this close to your surgery date. And consider showering with *antimicrobial soap*, paying special attention to wash the areas to be operated on. This will help prepare those areas for surgery. Make sure you get plenty of rest the evening before surgery, as well, even though you will no doubt be almost too excited to sleep.

Remember, no food or drink, except water, after midnight. Why is this important? If you have eaten just prior to surgery, it is possible that the contents of your stomach could come up, causing choking. Or you could inhale food particles into your lungs, causing a condition known as aspiration pneumonia.

I am so much smaller on top now after my breast reduction. Most people think I have lost weight. The change is dramatic. No more back pain. I can buy clothes that fit.

— Alicia, 31

The Day of Your Procedure

Your surgeon will likely give you instructions to follow. Those instructions will probably include some of the following.

Bathing

You'll probably want to take advantage of the fact that you are allowed to bathe on the day of your surgery, because you won't be able to shower for a few days after your procedure. So, feel free to bathe the day of, but remember that you cannot use any products, such as oils, lotions, make up—not even deodorant. Again, make sure you wash your surgical areas with antimicrobial soap to cleanse your body and prepare it for your procedure.

Remove Nail Polish

You'll also need to remove nail polish from at least one of your fingernails on each hand so that your medical team can monitor the color of your nails and ensure that your blood is well oxygenated during surgery. A probe that measures the amount of oxygen in blood also will be placed on your finger before surgery.

No Food Today

Remember, no food or liquids today. If your surgeon makes an exception and allows you to continue to take your current medication on the day of your procedure, take the tiniest sip of water possible with it. And when you are brushing your teeth, remember not to swallow any water while rinsing your mouth.

What to Wear

Choose function over form. Wear loose-fitting clothing that opens in the front. Be comfortable right down to your toes by wearing shoes that can be slipped off easily. Make sure you leave the jewelry at home today.

Questions to Ask Your Surgeon on How to Prepare for Your Procedure:

- What kind of pregnancy test will I be required to take? When?

- Do you need a letter from my general practitioner or OB/GYN giving me clearance for surgery?

- Do I need a mammogram?

- What method do you recommend that I use to quit smoking, since I'm not allowed to use any kind of nicotine replacement?

CHAPTER FIVE

Your Surgical Procedure

5

Your Surgical Procedure

··

*T*he day for your surgery has arrived. As exciting as this day is, however, you may find yourself experiencing some anxiety about your procedure. This is normal. Although the thought of undergoing surgery is never without some degree of trepidation, sometimes it helps if you know beforehand exactly what the procedure entails. That way, you can mentally rehearse your surgery day and run through the steps in your head until you feel as prepared emotionally for your surgery as you do physically. Let's take some time to discuss what happens on the day of your surgery.

Arriving at the Surgical Center

Your surgery will take place either at a hospital or at a surgical center. Some patients prefer a surgical center to a hospital because of the privacy, intimacy, and comfort this setting can offer because of its small size. Regardless of your location, upon your arrival the day of your procedure, the medical staff will greet you and lead you into a patient room, where you will change into a hospital gown. You may be asked to undergo a urine pregnancy test to ensure that you have not become pregnant since the last time you were tested.

An *intravenous (IV)* line will be inserted into a vein in your arm or perhaps in the top of your hand. You will feel the prick of the needle. This IV line will be used to deliver anesthesia and all other medications needed during your surgery.

How Long Will You Be at the Surgery Center?

You can expect to spend the better part of the day here. On average, your procedure will take approximately ninety minutes to three hours. The more breast tissue and fat you are having removed, the longer your surgery will take.

Once your surgery is completed, you'll be in a recovery room until you are awake and alert. If your surgery is to be an out-patient procedure, the medical staff will want to make sure your vital signs are stable and that you are ready to be taken home.

Meeting Your Medical Team

Your surgeon will not work alone. A team consisting of several healthcare professionals will be involved in your surgery. This team will likely include an anesthesiologist, your plastic surgeon, a physician technician, and two or three nurses.

Just prior to your operation, you will meet with your *anesthesiologist*, who will outline the details of the anesthesia process and answer any questions you may have about it.

You'll also meet with your plastic surgeon, who will use a marking pen, much like a felt-tip pen, to draw lines on your body, showing where incisions will be made. The surgeon will make these marks while you are standing to make sure that both breasts will be symmetrical.

Once you've been wheeled into the operating room, you will be transferred to a narrow surgical table. You will be secured with straps that resemble seat belts.

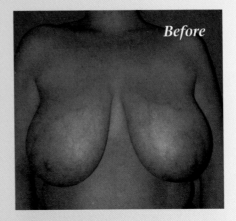

Before

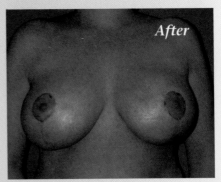

After

Age: 29. Procedure: Breast reduction
Tissue removed: 1.1 pound (500 grams) from each breast
Postoperative: Two weeks

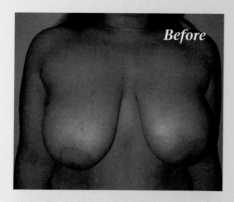

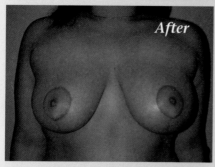

Age: 27. Procedure: Breast reduction
Tissue removed: 1.1 pound (500 grams)
from each breast
Postoperative: Three months

Compression Stockings

Just before you receive anesthesia, the medical team will put special *compression stockings* around your legs to improve circulation to your lower extremities while you're under anesthesia. These devices, technically known as *intermittent sequential compression devices* (SCDs), inflate and tighten much like a blood pressure cuff and are intended to prevent the formation of blood clots in the legs. Known as *deep vein thrombosis*, or DVT, such clots can travel to the heart or lungs and be fatal.

Receiving Anesthesia

Just prior to the surgery beginning, the anesthesiologist will administer *general anesthesia* through your IV. Within a minute or two, you will gently drift off to sleep. You will not feel any pain at this point. The anesthesiologist will monitor you throughout the procedure.

Monitoring Devices

A nurse will wrap a blood pressure cuff around your arm to monitor your blood pressure throughout the surgery. The nurse will also attach electrodes on your heart to ensure that your heartbeat remains regular throughout your procedure.

A pulse oximeter, a device typically clipped onto the forefinger, is an external probe that uses light bounced off the blood vessels under the probe to determine levels of "blood gases," or oxygenation of the hemoglobin in the blood cells.

Breathing Tube Insertion

Once you are asleep, your medical team will insert a breathing tube down your throat. The breathing tube is used to open and protect your airway and is connected to a breathing machine which will breathe for you while you're under anesthesia. You may notice that your throat feels a little sore after surgery from the breathing tube.

Breast Reduction Surgery

As part of the preparation for surgery, nurses will brush an antiseptic solution across your chest. This process will sterilize the skin's surface. The medical team will drape your body with cloth, leaving your breasts exposed. You'll be covered with a warm heating blanket, since operating rooms generally are kept quite chilly. Operating suites are cool because surgeons must perform procedures in "unbreathable" surgery gowns under very bright, powerful, hot lights. Also, cooler temperatures do not promote the growth of bacteria as well as warm environments.

Incision Techniques

Plastic surgeons have employed a variety of techniques to perform breast reduction surgery over the years. Today in the United States, the most popular breast reduction methods are the *anchor technique* and the *lollipop technique*. The type of incision used to perform the breast reduction will depend on the size and the droop of the breasts. In essence, the larger the breast, the larger the incisions will be.

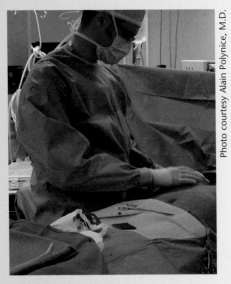

Photo courtesy Alain Polynice, M.D.

Breast reduction surgery, underway here, usually takes between two and four hours to complete.

Anchor Technique

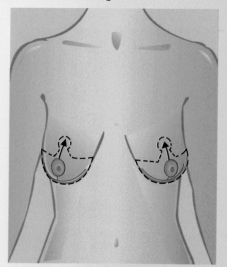

The anchor technique requires more incisions. The larger the breast, the more likely this type of incision will be needed.

The anchor technique incision also leaves a scar in the inframammary fold, or crease, of the breast.

The Anchor Technique

The anchor technique is the older of the two breast reduction techniques. It's called the anchor technique because the incisions are anchor-shaped. This approach is typically used with women who have greater amounts of tissue to be removed.

When executing the anchor technique, the surgeon removes excess breast tissue from the inner, upper and outer parts of the breast. Once the breast is shaped, all incisions are closed. The anchor method is considered what's called an *inferior-based pedicle technique,* because the nipple and areola remain attached to an island of breast tissue based inferiorly—on the lower portion of the breast.

The traditional anchor technique leaves horizontal scars, which run from under the breasts to the center of the chest; this scar may be from ten to twelve inches long. However, some surgeons use a newer variation on this technique, which leaves a horizontal scar that is only one to five inches long. This scar, which is under the breast, is hidden in the *inframammary fold.*

The anchor technique is not recommended if you are a woman of color prone to developing keloids, because the scarring is even more visible on darker shades of skin than it is on lighter skin.

The Lollipop Technique

This lollipop technique, also referred to as a *vertical technique,* received its name because the incision pattern resembles the shape of a lollipop. This approach is used for a woman who has smaller breasts. It leaves fewer scars than the anchor technique.

With this technique, the excess breast tissue is removed from the upper, outer, and lower parts of the breast. Usually, the lollipop technique includes a very small horizontal incision in the crease at the bottom of the breasts, but sometimes no horizontal incision is made. This smaller incision minimizes horizontal scarring. The lollipop technique is considered a *superior based* or *supero-medial-based pedicle technique* because the areola and nipple remain attached to an island of breast based superiorly, on the upper portion of the breast.

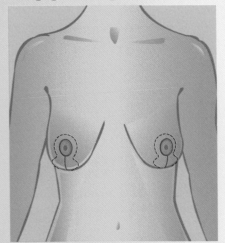

The incision used in the "lollipop technique" resembles a lollipop. In some cases, a horizontal incision is also required in the crease of the breast.

Breast Reduction

Procedure: Reduction mammoplasty

Length: 1.5 to 4 hours

Anesthesia: General anesthesia

In/Out Patient: Out-patient or short-term stay

Side Effects: Bruising, swelling, numbness, soreness, scars

Risks: Infection, asymmetry, loss of nipple sensation

Recovery: Initial: 7-10 days / Full: several months

Making Breasts Symmetrical

Your surgeon will complete most of the procedure on one breast and then repeat the same process on the other breast. He or she will not fully *suture* (stitch) your breasts at this time, however. Instead, he or she will tack together each breast at the corners. Although you will be lying flat for most of your procedure, at this point the surgeon will tilt you up to a sitting up position to ensure that your breasts look symmetrical when you are vertical, as well as horizontal.

Because many women naturally have one breast that is larger than the other, symmetry may not have been achieved at this point.

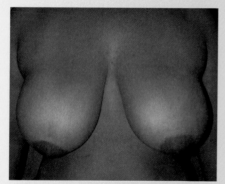

A 28-year-old woman with large breasts—38DDD cup.

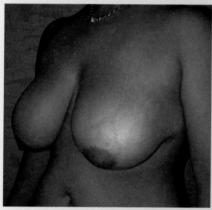

The large breasts cause back pain, bra strap furrowing at the shoulders, and rashes under the breasts.

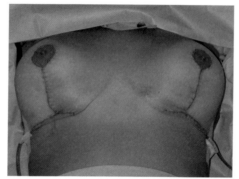

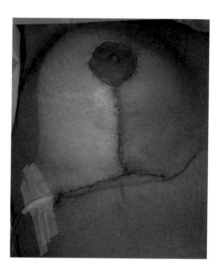

The same 28-year-old woman is shown immediately after breast reduction surgery.

Drainage tubes are held in place with Steri-Strips.

If any asymmetry is detected, your surgeon will make the necessary adjustments to make sure both breasts match as closely as possible until the proper balance is found.

During breast reduction surgery, surgeons commonly reduce the size of the areola. The size of a normal areola is one and a half to two inches; your surgeon will reduce the size of your areola to make it proportional to your new breast.

Inserting Drainage Tubes

Once your breasts are balanced, your surgeon will finalize the procedure by inserting *drainage tubes*. These drains are intended to prevent *hematomas*, the pooling of blood, and *seroma*, the pooling of serous fluid, or serum, after surgery. Serum, a clear fluid, is part of the blood.

Why is there a risk of fluids pooling? Any time the surgeon needs to move or pull the skin, it requires first separating the skin from the underlying tissue structures. This process is called *undermining*. Before the incision heals and the skin "re-adheres" to the underlying structures, a space is created. The body's fluids, mostly residual blood and serous fluid seep into this space. These fluids may not dissipate and may become infected. So, the drains must be left in place until fluid is no longer collecting under the skin.

The drain tubes themselves are small rubber tubes about three millimeters in diameter—thinner than a pencil. Rubber "bulbs" attached to the ends of the drainage tubes act as suction devices and gather excess blood and fluid.

Some surgeons insert these tubes into separate, tiny incisions. Other surgeons may secure the tube at the end of an incision. Your surgeon may secure the tubes with a suture or with Steri-Strips, commonly called "butterfly stitches." Steri-strips are pieces of surgical tape designed to hold together and protect incisions. Many patients prefer steri-strips because movement may cause the sutures to pull, creating discomfort. And sutures need to be removed in the doctor's office usually with slight discomfort. Steri-Strips, on the other hand are removed without any discomfort. After drainage tubes are inserted, your surgeon will suture your breasts using internal sutures and Steri-Strips externally. Note that some surgeons still use external sutures that need to be removed in the office.

The length of time you will need the drains depends on the quality and quantity of blood or fluid that drains from the incision site. You may need the drains for as little as two to three days or as long as two weeks. You will be responsible for monitoring the amount of fluid your drains capture and emptying them several times a day when they become full.

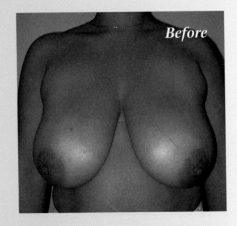

Before

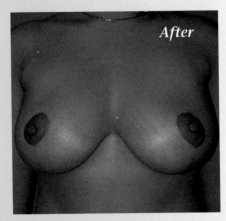

After

Age: 34. Procedure: Breast reduction
Tissue removed: 1.1 pounds (500 grams) from each breast
Postoperative: Three months

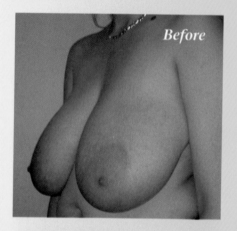

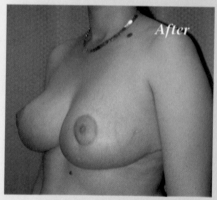

Age: 31. Procedure: Breast reduction
Tissue removed: 2.2 pounds (1,000 grams) from each breast
Postoperative: Six months

After Your Procedure

You will awaken immediately after your procedure is performed but will still be a little drowsy when you are transported to the recovery area. You'll be wearing a support garment designed to restrict your breasts' movement until they have begun to recover from your surgery. This garment is a Lycra/cotton bra that comfortably supports the breasts. Most likely, your surgeon will request that you stay at the hospital or surgical center for at least a couple of hours postsurgery for observation and to wait for your anesthesia to wear off. Remember, you will not be capable of driving a car immediately after surgery and will need to have made arrangements for someone you trust to drive you home and care for you for a couple of days.

Side Effects of Breast Surgery

All surgical procedures carry temporary side effects. These are normal and to be expected. Common side effects include:

- Soreness and discomfort, particularly at and near the incision sites.
- Numbness. Some nerves will be affected during surgery. This may cause temporary numbness; it usually disappears within four months.
- Bruising, which is very common when your skin is being stretched and pulled. Much of the bruising will fade during the first two weeks.
- Swelling, particularly around the incision sites. Swelling will diminish significantly during the first few weeks but can take months to fully resolve.

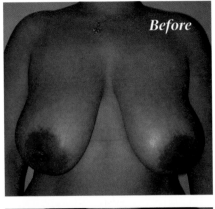
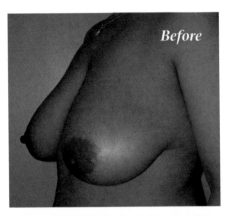
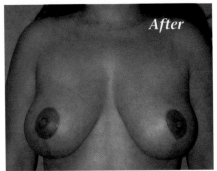
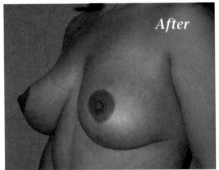

Age: 30. Procedure: Breast reduction

Tissue removed: Just under 1 pound (400 grams) from each breast
Postoperative: Three months

I had pain the first two days after breast reduction surgery. I used the pain medications. After that, the pain dissipated. I am very happy with my result.

— Sarah, 36

- Scarring, which is unavoidable. Initially scars will turn brighter red and purple before fading. It will take a full year for scars to fade and blend with your natural skin color. They may continue to fade thereafter, but they will never disappear completely.
- Low mood. You may find feel somewhat depressed the first week after surgery. This may be caused by a number of factors. There is usually an emotional "let down" after the surgery is finally over. Also, anesthesia may be a factor in your feeling down. At the same time, the fact that you are restricted from moving around vigorously is another factor. This type of temporary post-operative depression is quite normal.

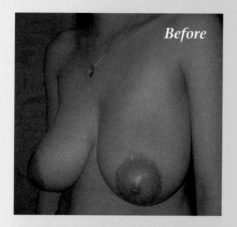

Before

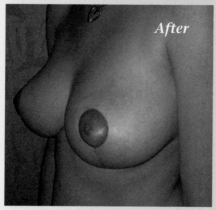

After

Age: 29. Procedure: Breast reduction
Tissue removed: 1.4 pounds (650 grams)
from each side
Postoperative: One year

Risks and Possible Complications of Breast Surgery

It is important to balance your enthusiasm for the new shape you soon will have with the recognition that every surgical procedure involves some serious issues to consider prior to the operation. Part of your surgeon's job is to inform you of these factors while you're deciding whether or not breast surgery is right for you. The chance of breast surgery complications is unlikely, but still, it's always good to be an informed consumer.

Allergic Reaction or Infection

There's a slim chance you'll experience an adverse reaction to anesthesia during surgery or acquire some sort of infection afterward. The American Society of Plastic Surgeons (ASPS) reports that an estimated 1 to 2 percent of breast reduction patients develop some sort of infection after surgery.

Delayed Healing

The ASPS reports that up to 21 percent of all breast reduction patients experience some form of delayed healing, ranging in severity from minor wound separation to actual skin loss. Usually, this condition is treatable. Patients most at risk for delayed healing include smokers, diabetics, obese people, and the elderly.

The size of the scar can influence delayed healing. There is a decreased incidence of delayed healing in patients whose breast reduction surgery involved techniques that use shorter incisions.

Loss of Nipple Sensation

It's possible that you could encounter a loss of circulation if a large amount of tissue and fat is removed, although it is unlikely. Some amount of nipple loss from this condition occurs in approximately 4 percent of breast reduction patients, according to the ASPS. Another risk relates to a lessening of nipple sensation. It's good to know, however, that if you do experience a decrease in nipple sensation, it usually returns fully within a year after surgery. There is, however, a slight possibility that you could be one of an estimated 13 percent (ASPS) of women who undergo breast surgery and report a permanent increase or decrease in nipple sensation. Pigment changes in the breast area have also been reported.

Breast Asymmetry and Shape Complications

Nearly all breast reduction patients experience some sort of discrepancy in size and shape of their breasts after surgery. Remember, though, that this is usually subtle and not much different from the slight irregularities that exist in most women naturally. Because breasts are "living canvases," plastic surgeons cannot guarantee that your final results will be perfectly symmetrical. Only about 5 percent of breast reduction patients experience asymmetry or shape irregularities significant enough to undergo an additional corrective surgery, according to the ASPS.

Fat Necrosis

Rarely, during the first few days after surgery, some of the fatty breast tissue dies because it receives insufficient blood flow. This can occur anywhere inside the breast, and once this tissue dies, it hardens, like scar tissue. You can feel it when you touch your breast. The ASPS estimates that 2 percent of breast reduction patients experience this complication. This condition will likely dissipate over the next few months as the tissues naturally soften. Breast massage may speed the

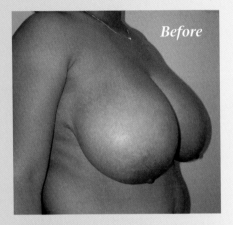

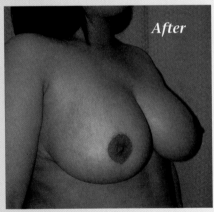

Age: 29. Procedure: Breast reduction
Tissue removed: 1.7 pounds (750 grams) from each side
Postoperative: Six months

I had breast reduction a year ago. My nipples were numb at first, but the sensation is now returning. My surgeon tells me I will be able to breastfeed if I so choose.

— *Christina, 29*

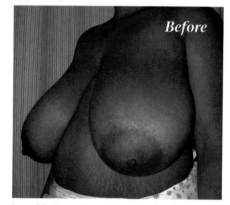 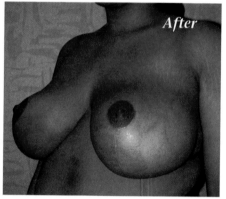

Age: 31. Procedure: Breast reduction

Tissue removed: 4.2 pounds (1,900 grams) from each side
Postoperative: Three months

process along. If the hardened tissue does not resolve, your surgeon may remove it with a minor surgical procedure.

Hemotoma and Seroma

A *hematoma* is the pooling of blood under the skin's surface. A *seroma* is a related complication. It is caused by excessive serum under the skin; serum is the clear fluid portion of blood.

The pooling of blood or fluid can put pressure on the inside of the skin and interfere with circulation, causing the skin to deteriorate. These conditions are more common when extremely large breasts are reduced, but are rare and would almost never go unnoticed.

If a small hematoma or seroma does develop, it may need to be drained. If so, you would need to return to the operating room, where your surgeon would open a few of the sutures and allow the accumulated blood or fluid to be drained out. In more extreme cases, skin is repaired with reconstructive surgery. The drainage tubes used in breast reduction surgery greatly diminish the risk of developing these conditions. According to the ASPS, hematomas occur in approximately 4 percent of breast reduction patients, and seromas develop in around 1 to 2 percent. Most of the time, these conditions begin to surface within the forty-eight hours after surgery.

Hardening of Tissue

It's also possible that you may experience a temporary hardening of the tissue around and underneath the nipple, but this condition should correct itself with massages and the natural softening of the scars. Breast tenderness during the first six months after surgery also is common.

Scarring

A reality of breast surgery is scarring. But, thanks to modern techniques, it's been minimized quite a bit in recent years. Most scars become unnoticeable in time, but some people may have a tendency to develop thick or hypertrophic scars or even keloids. People prone to keloids (fleshy tumors—large masses of scars) may want to avoid any kind of surgery altogether. The ASPS reports that 2 to 10 percent of breast reduction patients suffer from "abnormally heavy scars."

Healing after Surgery

The final result of your breast surgery won't be visible for several months. So, don't judge the success of your surgery on how your breasts look in the days immediately following your procedure. You will have bruising and swelling. The bruises will be red or purple initially, and will turn green and yellow as you heal. Initially, your

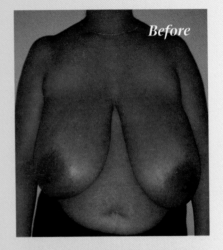

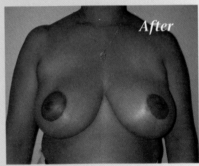

Age: 35. Procedure: Breast reduction
Tissue removed: 3.9 pounds (1,750 grams) from each side
Postoperative: Six months

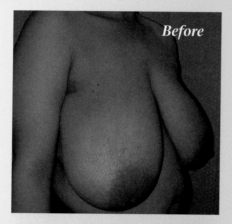

Before

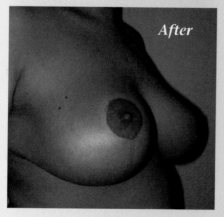

After

Age: 32. Procedure: Breast reduction
Tissue removed: 1.6 pounds (750 grams) from each side
Postoperative: Six months

breasts may have a "boxy" appearance, or they may appear somewhat cone-shaped. You may even see some rippling along the incisions, but these side effects will dissipate over a period of months. Your breasts will take on a more shapely appearance as they heal.

How quickly does the healing process occur? This will vary with each individual; however, there are three stages of healing. The first stage is known as the *inflammatory phase*, which usually lasts three to seven days. During this time, the incision site is swollen, may feel warm to the touch, and is quite red; this color will last for several weeks.

The second phase of healing, known as the *metabolic phase*, lasts for several weeks. During this time, the body is building new tissues to strengthen the incision site. During this phase, the body's healing mechanisms often produce scars that are somewhat thick; however, these scars will diminish later, during the third stage of healing, known as the *remodeling phase*. This is the time during which the body will "remodel" the scar. The collagen that has developed becomes stronger, and tissues become more elastic. The incision site becomes smaller and flatter. The color of the scar begins to fade, and the scar becomes less thick.

It may take as long one to two years before an incision is totally healed. Such things as smoking and vitamin deficiencies can impair healing.

A Word about Breastfeeding

You may be wondering whether breastfeeding is a possibility after breast surgery. A lot of confusion seems to surround this topic. Breastfeeding should still be a likely possibility for you. There is a good chance, however, that you may produce less breast milk than you did prior to your surgery. You may need to supplement your breast milk with formula. Talk to your surgeon more about the specifics.

- Which technique will be used to perform my procedure?

- What are the risks of my procedure, and how common are they?

- How long will it take to perform my surgery?

- How much tissue will be removed?

- Will I need to have drainage tubes inserted?

- Will liposuction be used during my surgery?

- How much scarring can I expect?

- Should I be able to leave the hospital or surgical center a couple of hours after my procedure, or will I need to spend the night there for observation?

- Will I be able to effectively breastfeed after my surgery?

CHAPTER SIX

Breast Lifts

6

Breast Lifts

*I*t's often difficult for women to adjust to changes in breast shape. When sagging or drooping occurs, many women don't feel as attractive as they once did. They may wish to alter their breast size and form simply to feel better about themselves.

In you find yourself in this situation, you may be considering a breast lift. Unlike breast reduction, which is often a medical necessity, a breast lift if a purely cosmetic procedure.

What Is a Breast Lift?

A breast lift, also known as a *mastopexy*, is a procedure to remove excess skin and reshape the breast tissue in order to lift and support drooping breasts. The medical term for the sag or droop in the breasts is *ptosis* (pronounced: toe-sis). The degree of ptosis is classified according to the relationship between the nipple and the inframammary fold, the crease below the breast. In the normal breast, the nipple lies above the inframammary fold and on the mound of the breast. The degrees are ptosis are:

- First degree: minimal droop; the nipple lies at the level of the fold.
- Second degree: moderate droop; the nipple is below the fold but is still above the lowest part of the breast.
- Third degree: major droop; the nipple lies below the fold and at the lower part of the breast.
- Pseudoptosis: the nipple is above the inframammary fold, but the breast tissue falls below it.

Causes of Sagging

Whether breasts are large or small, ptosis is inevitable No one is immune to the effects of gravity. All females who live beyond adolescence will experience some degree of sagging during their lifetime.

The degree of ptosis, however, does vary from woman to woman. A variety of elements contribute to this difference, the most significant of which is breast size. Because breasts consist of only ligaments, fat, and connective tissue and do not contain any actual muscle, breasts begin to droop over time. The ligaments and skin lose their elasticity and begin to stretch.

Although ptosis is inevitable, the rate at which it occurs also is affected by genes, diet, aging, and breast size. Pregnancy, breastfeeding, and menopause contribute to ptosis, as well. Many childless women, however, also complain of drooping breasts. Ptosis is especially evident after significant weight loss.

Generally speaking, women with small breasts will not experience as much sagging as women with larger breasts. Women with smaller breasts have less breast tissue pulling the breasts down.

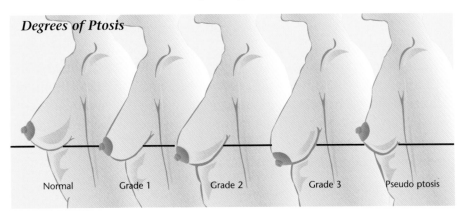

Degrees of Ptosis

Normal   Grade 1   Grade 2   Grade 3   Pseudo ptosis

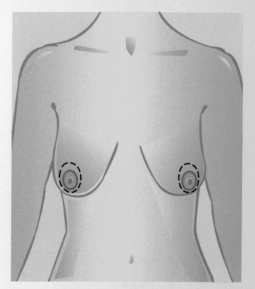

Most breast lifts are performed with the lollipop or anchor technique; however, some women with smaller breasts may have a "doughnut mastopexy," in which skin is removed from around the areola.

Are You a Candidate for a Breast Lift?

Maybe you are pleased with the size of your breasts but simply would like to have a shapelier, firmer, more youthful look. Or maybe you would even like to increase the size of your breasts or slightly decrease them just a little. If this is your situation and you are in overall good health, you are probably a good candidate for a breast lift.

However, if you plan to have children in the future, you may want to wait until after your last pregnancy before having this procedure. Another pregnancy could reverse your surgical results, and further ptosis may occur in the future.

How Is a Breast Lift Performed?

The same basic incision techniques are used for breast lifts and reductions. Many women who want only a breast lift with no reduction are candidates for the lollipop technique, which will leave less scaring. The surgeon's approach will depend, in part, on the degree of droop in your breasts. In cases involving lesser degrees of sagging, a *circumareolar incision*, which is made around the areola, only may be used. This technique is also called a *doughnut mastopexy*. Drainage tubes are not typically utilized during breast lifts that include augmentation.

In order to shape an attractive breast mound during a breast lift, the surgeon may also need to remove some breast tissue. The major difference between a breast reduction and a breast lift is the amount of tissue removed during surgery. As mentioned earlier, a procedure is considered a breast lift and not a breast reduction if less than 500 grams of fat and breast tissue is removed.

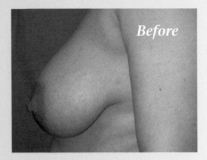

Before

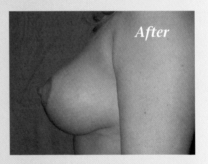

After

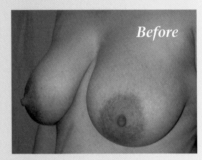

Before

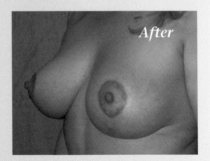

After

> ### *Breast Lift*
>
> **Procedure:** Mastopexy / lifts and reshapes breasts
>
> **Length:** 1.5 to 3 hours
>
> **Anesthesia:** General anesthesia or local with sedation
>
> **In/Out Patient:** Out-patient or short-term in-patient
>
> **Side Effects:** Bruising, swelling, soreness, scars.
>
> **Risks:** Infection, asymmetry, loss of nipple sensation
>
> **Recovery:** Initial: 7 to 10 days / Full: several months

Breast Lift with Augmentation

For some women, a breast lift alone corrects sagging and produces a shapely breast. However, there are times when removing excess skin and lifting the breast will not produce a shapely breast. These are cases in which a woman is lacking sufficient breast tissue to produce an attractive breast mound. If this is your situation, your plastic surgeon will likely recommend an implant, or augmentation, along with the breast lift.

Types of Implants

If you are considering a breast lift with augmentation, you'll need to have a dialogue about this with your surgeon. He or she will create an augmentation plan individually catered to meet your needs. Implants now come in a variety of shapes, sizes, and textures.

Age: 32. Procedure: Breast lift
Postoperative: Six months

I had little pain after my breast lift. I was sore, but I didn't need to take the pain medications. My scars healed nicely, too.

— *Dawn, 29*

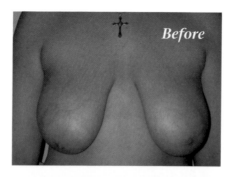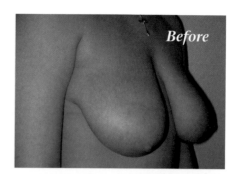

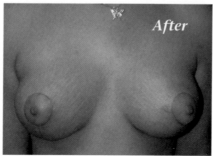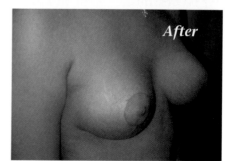

Age: 20. Procedure: Breast lift   Postoperative: Three months

Saline Implants

The vast majority of implants used today are made of a soft silicone shell, filled with saline, which is saltwater. Medical professionals consider saline to be safe as an implant filler, because it consists only of salt and water—two ingredients that our bodies contain already; as a result, even if a leak should occur, the saline would easily be absorbed by the body.

Silicone Implants

Implants are filled with silicone gel. Many surgeons and women alike find that silicone implants have a more natural feel. However, FDA restrictions permit the use of silicone-gel implants only in controlled clinical studies for the purposes of reconstruction after mastectomy, correction of congenital deformities, or replacement of ruptured silicone-gel implants that were used for augmentation. Silicone implants can also be used in women with saline implants who have had either complications or problems and are unsatisfied.

You may recall hearing about the controversy in the 1990s over whether silicone implants are safe. Some women whose implants ruptured claimed the silicone made them ill. Leaks in silicone implants are not easily detected; however, years of studies have produced no hard data that connect silicone implants with disease.

Implant Shapes

Implants can be round or anatomical, which is a tear-drop shape. Most women prefer round implants to anatomical ones, because they give a fuller appearance. Some implants are called high-profile implants—they project farther out from the chest and may be best suited for women with small chests and narrow frames.

Implant Texture

Implants come in either smooth or textured surfaces. Smooth implants can move freely in the "pocket" created for them, and many women report the smooth shell surface make the implant less detectable to the touch on the breast's exterior. Textured implants, which do not move freely, were designed to lessen the risk of capsular contracture; however, studies vary on whether they do this. Some women believe the textured surface does not feel as natural through the skin as the round implants. Today, most women choose smooth implants.

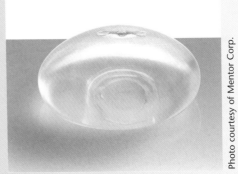

Photo courtesy of Mentor Corp.

The round, smooth implant is most commonly used in breast augmentation surgery.

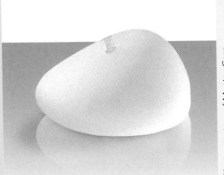

Photo courtesy of Mentor Corp.

The textured implant, in the same shape of a tear drop, is an alternative style of implant.

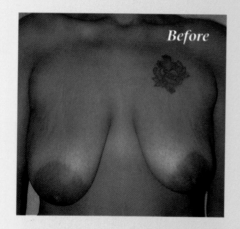

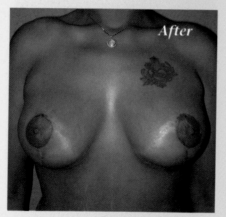

Age: 35. Woman with asymetrical breasts
Procedure: Breast lift with augmentation
Implants: 280 cc on left, 175 cc on right
Postoperative: Four weeks

Implant Size

Breast implants are measured in cubic centimeters (cc). Most implants used in general range in size between 125cc and 700cc. In recent years, women have been choosing larger implants than they did previously. Surgeons will not typically approve implants that would yield an unnatural appearance on patients, though. Your body type, height, and weight all must factor into which size will best meet your needs. You and your surgeon will work together to find the perfect size for you. He or she may even ask you to experiment with different sizes by wearing them in your bra or under a T shirt during the consultation.

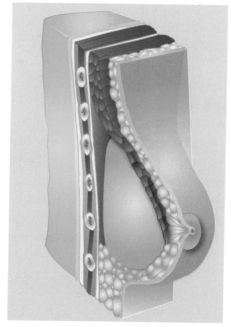

Submuscular placement of the implant.

Placement of Implants

During your consultation, you and your surgeon will discuss the best type of implant for you and exactly where your implants will be placed. Factors that determine implant placement include your breast shape and basic anatomy, breast tissue amount, general size of your body, and your favorite exercise activities.

Submuscular Placement

Most often, surgeons prefer to insert implants partially under the pectoral muscles. The advantages to this placement: a more natural look, edges of the implant are less likely to be noticed, rippling is less likely, and there is a lower risk of a complication known as a *capsular contracture*. A capsular contracture occurs when scar tissue forms around the implants. Another important advantage of submuscular placement is that there is no interference with mammograms.

Disadvantages are that the implants may create more of an upper roundness in the breasts than you'd like; there is also more postoperative discomfort. Implants placed under the muscle wall usually cause some discomfort which can last for seven to ten days after surgery, because pectoral muscles are in the process of stretching over the implants. Usually, the discomfort is worse for women who have not had children. Why? Because their breast tissues are usually tighter. This discomfort, however, often improves somewhat within forty-eight hours after surgery.

Note that your implants may appear to "ride" high within the first few weeks after surgery. This is common. They should drop to a more pleasing position after the swelling subsides and the implants settle into place.

Subglandular Placement

A subglandular placement means the implant is placed behind the breast tissue and in front of the pectoral muscle. The advantages to this placement are that the

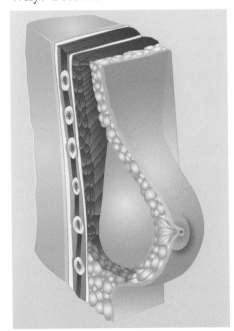

Subglandular placement of the implant.

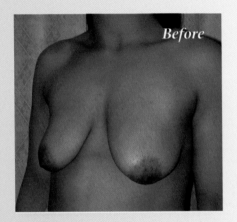

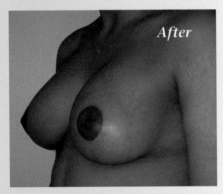

Age: 22. Procedure: Breast lift with implants
Implants: 300 cc
Postoperative: Three months

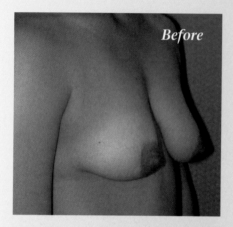

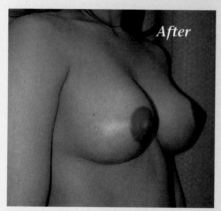

Age: 29. Procedure: Breast lift with implants
Implants: 275 cc
Postoperative: One year

implants are easier for the surgeon to insert, there is less discomfort and shorter recovery time, and larger implants can be inserted. The disadvantages are that ripples in the skin are more likely and capsular contracture is more likely.

Are You a Candidate for Breast Lift with Augmentation?

As with any breast lift or reduction, you may want to wait until you have completed your family before committing to a breast lift with augmentation. Implants have not been proven to interfere with pregnancy or breastfeeding, but it's a strong possibility that your breasts will sag as they did prior to surgery, even with implants, if you experience another pregnancy later.

Other candidates for breast lifts with augmentation are women whose breasts are noticeably different sizes. Surgeons insert an implant only in the smaller breast, to create a more balanced appearance. Basically, if you desire larger, firmer, or fuller breasts, a breast lift with implants may be a desirable choice for you.

If you are considering a breast lift with augmentation, a factor to consider is that your breasts will not feel as natural with implants as they do without them. Instead, you will notice that your breasts are rounder and firmer than they were before, which a lot of women actually are pleased about. In fact, you may not even need to wear a bra after having your implants inserted.

Breast Lift with Augmentation Procedure

The surgical procedure of a breast lift with augmentation is similar to that of the basic breast lift. The incision made for a breast lift with augmentation is often lollipop-shaped; however, if a woman has severe sagging, the anchor-shaped incisions may be necessary.

Risks and Complications of Breast Lift with Augmentation

As with any surgery, certain risks and complications apply to breast lifts with augmentation, as well. In addition to the risks associated with traditional breast lifts, breast lifts that include implant insertion could potentially cause a condition called capsular contracture. This situation occurs when the scar or the capsule surrounding the implant begins to tighten, causing the breast to feel hard. Capsular contracture is rectified either by removing the implant or operating on the breast's scar tissue.

Additional complications sometimes associated with breast augmentation include the formation of calcium deposits and implant shifting. Some women who've undergone silicone implant insertion have complained of immune system disorder symptoms, such as joint pain, swelling, fever, fatigue, and pain; however, no evidence has been found to support the hypothesis that implants actually caused these symptoms. Many studies have shown that women who do experience these symptoms may very well have developed them over time, even if their surgery were never performed.

Do Implants Affect Mammograms?

Although saline implants are not thought to be dangerous, you need to be aware that you will need to rely on radiologists who know how to X-ray patients with breast implants when you have mammograms. Implants, though not proven to cause breast cancer, appear white on mammograms and sometimes can block masses behind them. This is a problem associated with subglandular implants rather than submuscular implants.

This is not a concern, however, if various angles of your breasts are X-rayed by a radiologist with applicable experience. Make sure that

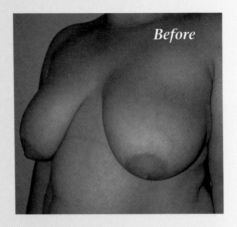

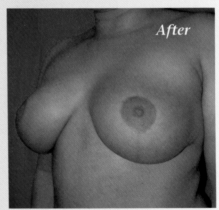

Age: 22. Procedure: Breast lift
Postoperative: Three months

After having children, my breasts were like deflated balloons. The sagged to my navel. It was traumatic. I was ashamed. After a breast lift, it was WOW! My breasts were normal again. It changed my life. I feel sexy again.

— Karen, 29

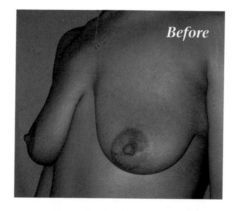 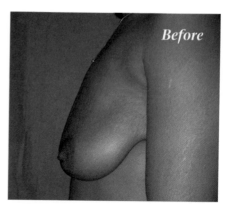

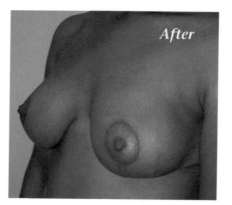 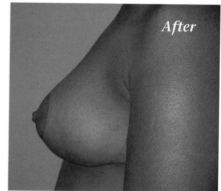

Age: 29. Procedure: Breast lift

Postoperative: One year

you inform the radiologist as well as the technician performing the study that you have had implants inserted before they complete the mammogram. If you desire a more sensitive method of breast cancer screening, you may wish to consider an MRI, which uses magnetic fields instead of radiation to screen for breast masses.

Paying for a Breast Lift

Insurance companies traditionally pay only for procedures that are medically necessary. As you realize, breast lifts are cosmetic. So the chances are not good for getting your insurance company to pay for a breast lift.

Questions to Ask Your Surgeon about Your Breast Lift:

- Which technique will you be using for my lift?

- What results can I realistically expect?

- Do I have enough breast tissue for a regular lift, or would you recommend implants, as well?

- Which size and shape of implants do you recommend for me?

- Will my implants be placed beneath the breast tissue or under the pectoral muscles?

- Will I need to have my implants removed someday?

CHAPTER SEVEN

Follow-up Care

7

Follow-up Care

our surgery is now behind you. You've made it through the most challenging part of the process and are now on the road to a healthier and happier you. Relax and take good care of yourself. Carefully attending to the healing stage is imperative to ensure that your surgery results come as close as possible to matching the image of yourself you've envisioned.

As with all women, your situation and your surgery are unique, and your surgeon will provide you with an individualized recovery program. During the next several weeks, you'll want to follow these recommendations to achieve optimal results. Still, there are basic guidelines for what you can expect after breast surgery.

What to Expect

Upon your arrival home, your breasts will be bruised and swollen; however, you won't notice this too much, because your breasts will still be secured by your surgical support garment for the next few days. You can expect your breasts to remain bruised for seven to ten days and swollen for four to six weeks.

Will I be in Pain?

It's likely that your anesthesia will not have fully worn off by the time you get home, so you should not be feeling any pain. Will you have pain in the days ahead? It is difficult to predict. Many patients report only mild discomfort after surgery and during the recovery period; others will have post-surgical pain for which they need pain medication. If this is the case, it's important to take pain medication prescribed by your surgeon.

Sometimes, patients decide to discontinue their pain medication if they are not feeling any discomfort, thinking that they no longer need it. This practice is not advisable, however, because often the medication masks pain, and pain flares up once the medication is stopped. To avoid the undesirable condition of "chasing pain," it's preferable "stay ahead" of the pain by taking your pain medication as recommended by your surgeon.

Usually, your surgeon will prescribe pain medication to be taken every four hours for one to two days, whether or not you are feeling any discomfort at the time. Beyond the first couple of days after your procedure, your surgeon most likely will recommend you take your pain medication whenever you begin to feel a twinge of discomfort.

A concern many patients have about pain medication is becoming addicted to it. If you take your pain medication in the dosage prescribed at the recommended intervals, though, you should not become vulnerable to addiction. Addiction to prescription drugs occurs only when patients take more than the recommended dosage or continue with medication longer than is medically necessary.

Will I Need Antibiotics?

Most likely, your surgeon will prescribe an *antibiotic* for you to take in addition to your pain medication while you are healing from your procedure. An antibiotic definitely will be used during your surgery to ensure that no infection develops, and your surgeon probably will recommend that you take one for approximately five days after your surgery. After your procedure, especially if you had drainage tubes inserted, your surgeon will most likely prescribe a course of antibiotics to prevent infection.

Emptying Drains

You will be responsible for emptying your own drains until your surgeon removes your drainage tubes at your first follow-up session, three to five days after surgery. A slim possibility is that your drains may still be gathering too much liquid for your surgeon to feel comfortable removing your tubes during the first follow-up session. If this is the case, he or she simply will schedule another session for you a few days later to remove them.

Emptying your drains should not be painful. You simply will need to be mindful to empty them as they become full. Even if your drains are not completely full, your surgeon probably will request that you empty them twice a day and record the amount of fluid they contain at those times.

Also, you will not be able to take a shower until twenty-four hours after your surgeon removes your drainage tubes at your first follow-up session. You may, however, take "sponge baths" during the first few days after your procedure.

Surgical Dressings

After your operation, your surgeon will have wrapped your breasts in a *surgical dressing*. These bandages will be covered by your surgical support garment and will not be your responsibility to change. You will leave the dressing alone for the first few days following surgery, and then your surgeon will evaluate your healing progress during your first follow-up session. During this process, your surgeon will remove your surgical garment, unwrap your dressing, and examine your new breasts. This will be the first time that you and your surgeon will be able to view the results of your procedure. Remember, your breasts still will appear swollen and bruised, but you should be able to glimpse the essence of your new look.

Your actual scars will not be visible at this time, however, because your Steri-Strips will still be in place. The Steri-Strips will fall off by themselves after you start showering. Once your surgeon evaluates your healing, he or she will change your dressings and replace your surgical support bra.

After your drainage tubes are removed, you may experience some light bleeding at the drainage tube sites for twenty-four hours or so; your surgeon may cover this area with a small gauze dressing. Twenty-four hours after your drainage tubes are removed, you may shower. Beyond that, no further dressing should be needed. Your surgeon will schedule a second follow-up session for you approximately two weeks after the first one to make sure you are continuing to heal properly.

Support Garments

Once you have worn your surgical support garment for three to four weeks after your procedure, you'll be free to choose a more comfortable support bra or Lycra sports bra to replace it. You will need to wear this kind of bra for the next four to six weeks to give your breasts the support they need to properly heal. You should not wear regular bras, especially underwires, because they could interfere with healing. Underwire bras, especially, can continually rub against your incisions under your breasts and irritate them. This could reopen your wounds. You may wash your surgical support bra or your Lycra bra as often as you need to.

Sutures

You don't need to worry about having sutures removed. Today most surgeons use internal, absorbable sutures. As mentioned earlier, your surgeon may cover your incisions with Steri-Strips.

My drains were left in for four days. I went back to work in about a week. I was sore, but didn't have a lot of post-op pain.

— Christina, 29

$\mathcal{M}$y breast reduction was an out-patient procedure. I was at the hospital most of the day, but went home that night.

— Allison, 36

Recovery at Home

Your initial recovery time will be seven to ten days. Your body needs time to heal. It's extremely important to heed your surgeon's advice about when to resume your daily routine. If you become too active too soon, you could open up your stitches and cause excessive bleeding. This could be dangerous and would delay your healing significantly.

You should be able to perform nonstrenuous daily activities, such as cooking, right away. You will not, however, be able to perform anything strenuous. And yes, driving your kids to school is considered strenuous after surgery. Avoid lifting heavy objects. You will be restricted from exercise of any kind for the first two weeks.

You can expect to resume moderate activity, such as vacuuming or driving, after your first seven to fourteen days after the operation. You'll be able to go back to work (assuming your job does not involve any kind of extreme physical labor) two weeks after your surgery. Around this time, it should be safe for you to resume sexual activity, as well.

Your complete recovery time will be approximately four to six weeks. Your plastic surgeon will advise you about the appropriate time to resume routine activities without restriction, including going to the gym and exercising.

Avoid the Sun

You should, however, wait at least six months until you intentionally expose your body to the sun at all, and wait one entire year before exposing your scars to sunlight, as in sunbathing or going to a tanning salon. Sun exposure too early can interfere with healing and cause scarring to appear more extreme. Because sun rays can reach your skin beneath your bathing suit, you will need to wear a sunscreen of at least SPF 15 on your scars beneath your bathing suit for at least one year.

Breast Massage

Another aspect of your healing requires your active participation. Within two to four weeks after your procedure, you will need to begin massaging the areas on your breasts where you see scars. Choose your favorite lotion—maybe one with cocoa butter as a major ingredient—and gently massage your breasts around the nipples and other scarred areas. You will need to do this for an entire year in order to significantly decrease your visible scarring. It sounds like a lot of work, but soon giving yourself a daily massage will become as routine as brushing your teeth. And it will all be worth it when your scars feel soft and fade quickly.

Touch-up Surgery

Touch-ups are not usually necessary with breast surgery. It's rare that breast procedures yield any undesirable effects that would require additional surgeries to be performed. It is, however, possible. Rarely, after surgery it is noted that a patient's breasts are uneven, as breasts often are naturally. In this situation, a surgeon may use liposuction to balance the breasts. Very rarely, a small revision surgery actually may be necessary. Usually, a revision can be done under local anesthesia.

Another issue that very rarely develops after surgery, but can require a touch-up, is a condition called hypertrophic scars, or "keloids." If keloids do develop, surgeons often try other forms of treatment before operating on them, because keloids often grow back after surgery.

If a touch-up surgery is required for whatever reason, usually it is free of cost for the patient, especially if both surgeon and patient agree that an improvement needs to be made. Ordinarily, patients are responsible for only the anesthesia and the surgical center charge if a touch-up is needed, although this practice may not be universal. Be sure to discuss this issue with your surgeon before committing to surgery.

Questions to Ask Your Surgeon

- How long is the recovery period?
- What kind of postoperative self-care will be necessary?
- When can I go back to work and resume other normal activities?
- What medication shall I take for post-operative pain management? How long?
- What is the procedure for emptying my drain?
- When can I take a shower again?
- When is my first post-surgical appointment?
- When is it safe to drink alcohol, smoke, take products containing aspirin, or be exposed to the sun again?
- When can I resume sexual activity?
- When can I wear regular bras again?
- How shall I perform my daily breast massage to decrease scarring?
- Will I need a touch-up surgery?

CHAPTER EIGHT

The New You!

8

The New You!

Having breast reduction surgery is a two-part journey. One part physical. One part emotional. Once your surgery is complete, you begin to heal physically. At the same time, you will likely begin to heal the emotional scars created over the years as you have suffered with large breasts.

Our old attitudes and beliefs don't change overnight, but you have taken a step that will produce dramatic changes in your life. You will feel some of the changes immediately. Others may come about more gradually. Give yourself credit for taking steps that help you lead a fuller, more active life. And most important, enjoy the journey.

What to Say to Others

You may or may not be self-conscious about discussing your breast surgery with others. You may wish to ponder what you're comfortable telling people when they comment on a change in your appearance. A lot of people will notice that you appear different somehow, but will not be able to put their finger on what exactly has been altered. If you've had a breast reduction or lift, many people will probably tell you that you appear thinner and ask what your weight loss secret is. You'll need to decide whether you will inform them of your procedure or refer them to the latest diet plan.

Your decision probably will be based on how well you know someone and whether they need to know. For example, you will probably want to inform your employer of your procedure, because you will need to miss some work. But whether you speak to him or her in general or specific terms about your procedure is your decision. What to say to friends and family will also be at your discretion. Really, it depends on your comfort level and what feels right to you.

Meet Your New Body

Your transformation will likely be most apparent first on the physical level. If you've had a breast reduction performed, once you've healed, you will feel lighter, move more freely, and find yourself standing taller. If you suffered from back, neck, and shoulder pain due to your breast size in the past, it should disappear the moment the extra weight is removed. Many women are surprised at how immediately their symptoms are relieved.

New Clothes

Women who have undergone breast surgery will soon realize that clothes now fit them very differently than they used to. These women should feel much better proportioned than they did before, and mixing and matching clothing sizes to find an outfit that fits should be a frustration of the past. The shopping you will need to do as a result of your new breast size and shape will be fun! And you'll be looking for more than just new bras. You will find that many of your old clothes just don't fit quite right—they are loose across your chest, or maybe the cut seems off.

You'll want to ask yourself what different types of clothing you'd like to explore now that you've acquired a new shape. Which garments did you avoid, even when they caught your eye across department store aisles, because you didn't have the confidence that you could

I bought a new coat recently. I couldn't believe I could easily find one that would fit. Prior to breast reduction, clothes that would fit across my chest would be way too big in the waist.

— Rebecca, 34

wear them? A dress with spaghetti straps, maybe? A new swimsuit, perhaps? No, breast surgery won't change your entire body, but if you're like most women, you will be pleased with your new look.

Meet Your New Sense of Self

That self-assured woman within you finally is able to show you how fun life can be. She's ready to go on that date now. She's signing up for a tap-dancing class. She even thinks she may want to give aerobics a try. Maybe she'll even go for a jog tomorrow! Sometimes it's hard to remember what got in the way of this active lifestyle before. But, really, it is difficult to completely forget the past and all of the obstacles you've overcome to reach this point.

Healing from a Painful Past

Chances are that you, like many other women who are uncomfortable with their breasts, avoided activities that others enjoy. Maybe you even hid under your clothing, wearing more than one bra or multiple layers of shirts. Perhaps you learned to sit with rounded shoulders to minimize the size of your breasts.

Because you've actually followed through with a breast surgery procedure, various motivating factors must have contributed to your decision. Some of these motivators may be rooted in deep emotional scars from years of being the subject of your peers' taunting and teasing. You may have even had a few humiliating experiences with significant others over the issue of your breasts. Or maybe for you it was subtler—that sinking feeling of dissatisfaction when you looked at yourself in the mirror.

Moving toward a Brighter Future

Hopefully, you'll find that these layers of self-consciousness surrounding your breasts that took many years to build are slowly beginning to dissolve now that you've completed your procedure. It takes a while, though, and it's normal to still have some of the old pain of the past rear its head from time to time. Although a major source of those insecurities has been removed from your life, don't be surprised if many of its emotional effects remain for a while. You've been through a lot over the years, and may have a lot of hurt to work through still. That's okay. It's a process, not an event. You may consider finding a good therapist to help you process some of your painful memories and support you through this transition of adjusting to your new body.

You do not have to hide anymore. In reality, you never truly did. You are valuable and attractive whatever your breast size or shape, because *who you are* is much more important than how you look. The hope is that your breast surgery helps you discover this fact.

Empowerment

Another hope is that you will find the confidence to work toward and achieve goals for yourself that you did not think possible before. Changing your breast size and shape can feel really empowering, because you've noticed something you are dissatisfied with, created a plan to improve it, and now are reaping the rewards of your efforts. Let your breast procedure be the first step in generalizing this practice to the rest of your life. What else in your life do you wish were different? How do you wish that situation looked instead? What steps would you need to take in order for your wishes to become a reality?

Now, take the first step…and then the second….Once you realize the personal power you have to create a life worth living, the easier it will be for you to map out your goals and take steps to make them happen.

As I look back, I suffered psychologically more than I realized about my big breasts, especially when I was in school. Boys teased me. I feel like a new person after breast reduction. My breasts fit my body.

— Sarah, 35

Resources

American Society of Plastic Surgeons

444 East Algonquin Road • Arlington Heights, IL 60005
Phone: 847-228-9900; 888-4-PLASTIC;
888-475-2784 (Physician referrals)
www.plasticsurgery.org

The American Society of Plastic Surgeons (ASPS) is the largest plastic surgery specialty organization in the world. Founded in 1931, the society is composed of board-certified plastic surgeons who perform cosmetic and reconstructive surgery. The mission of ASPS is to advance quality care to plastic surgery patients by encouraging high standards of training, ethics, physician practice, and research in plastic surgery. The society advocates for patient safety, such as encouraging its members to operate in surgical facilities that have passed rigorous external review of equipment and staffing. The society works in concert with the Plastic Surgery Educational Foundation, founded in 1948, which supports research and educational programs for plastic surgeons. On the society's Web site are FAQs, a history of plastic surgery, a surgeon finder, capsule descriptions of procedures, patient profiles, a photo gallery, and cost information.

American Board of Plastic Surgery

Seven Penn Center
1635 Market Street, Suite 400 • Philadelphia, PA 19103-2204
Phone: 215-587-9322 • Fax: 215-587-9622
www.abplsurg.org

The mission of the American Board of Plastic Surgery is to promote safe, ethical, efficacious plastic surgery to the public by maintaining high standards for the education, examination, and certification of plastic surgeons as specialists and subspecialists. Primarily for physicians, the board's Web site includes FAQs explaining how doctors become board-certified and describing differences among licensure, certification, and accreditation.

Federation of State Medical Boards

Federation Place
400 Fuller Wise Road, Suite 300 • Euless, Texas 76039-3855
Phone: 817-868-4000
www.fsmb.org

The Federation of State Medical Boards of the United States, Inc., is a national organization comprised of the 69 medical boards of the United States, the District of Columbia, Puerto Rico, Guam, and the U.S. Virgin Islands. The mission is to be a leader in improving the quality, safety, and integrity of health care in the United States by promoting high standards for physician licensure and practice. FSMB operates the Federation Physician Data Center, a nationally recognized system for collecting, recording, and distributing to state medical boards and other appropriate agencies data on disciplinary actions taken against licensees by the boards and other governmental authorities.

Food and Drug Administration

5600 Fishers Lane • Rockville, MD 20857-0001
Phone: 888-INFO-FDA, 888-463-6332
www.fda.gov

The Food and Drug Administration (FDA), which oversees the safety of food, cosmetics, medicines, medical devices, and radiation-emitting products, also has a consumer friendly Website. It posts consumer updates, a directory for consumer and manufacturer calls and complaints, and links to other on-line FDA manuals and publications.

American Board of Medical Specialties

1007 Church Street, Suite 404 • Evanston, IL 60201-5913
Phone: 847-491-9091 • Fax: 847-328-3596
www.abms.org

The American Board of Medical Specialties (ABMS) is an organization of twenty-four approved medical specialty boards. The intent of the certification of physicians is to provide assurance to the public that those certified by an ABMS member board have successfully completed an approved training program and an evaluation process assessing their ability to provide quality patient care in the specialty. This Web site explains how specialists are trained and certified; it also offers a search feature for finding certified physicians.

eMedicine, Inc.

1004 Farnam Street, Suite 300 • Omaha, NE 68102
Phone: 402-341-3222
www.emedicine.com

Though created for an audience of health professionals, the eMedicine Web site includes informative descriptions of hundreds of procedures. Launched in 1996, the site is the most comprehensive source of information available free online about procedures, risks, side effects, anesthesia, preparation for surgery, follow-up, expectations, and other pertinent information. Nearly 10,000 physician authors and editors contribute to the eMedicine Clinical Knowledge Base, which contains articles on 7,000 diseases and disorders. The site also contains nearly 6,500 pages of patient information.

The U.S. National Library of Medicine

8600 Rockville Pike • Bethesda, MD 20894
www.nlm.nih.gov
www.nlm.nih.gov/medlineplus

The National Library of Medicine Web site indexes articles from more than 3,500 medical journals. The service is aimed primarily at scientists and health professionals; however, MEDLINEplus is written for consumers.

American Academy of Cosmetic Surgery

Cosmetic Surgery Information Service
737 North Michigan Avenue, Suite 820 • Chicago, IL 60611
Phone: 312-981-6760
www.cosmeticsurgery.org

Formed in 1985, the American Academy of Cosmetic Surgery represents practitioners of medical disciplines, including plastic and reconstructive surgery, general surgery, dermatology, ophthalmology, otorhinolaryngology, oral and maxillofacial surgery, and others. The AACS is the nation's largest organization representing cosmetic surgeons.

The Academy's purpose is to maintain a membership of medical and dental professionals who participate in postgraduate medical education opportunities, specifically in cosmetic surgery, so that the public is assured of receiving consistently high-quality medical and dental care.

The Academy's Web site offers assistance choosing and finding a surgeon, describes procedures and their risks, explains what to do before surgery, and helps you determine whether you're a good candidate for specific procedures.

The American Society for Aesthetic Plastic Surgery

11081 Winners Circle • Los Alamitos, CA 90720
Phone: 800-364-2147 or 562-799-2356
Fax: 562-799-1098
www.surgery.org

Founded in 1967, ASAPS is a professional organization of plastic surgeons certified by the American Board of Plastic Surgery, who specialize in cosmetic plastic surgery. The organization has 1,900 members in the U.S. and Canada, as well as corresponding members in many other countries. The Web site can help you find a surgeon and offers an "Ask an ASAPS Surgeon" feature, as well as news, updates, and consumer-oriented reports on surgical and nonsurgical procedures. The site also has a Find-a-Surgeon feature. You'll find numerous articles and procedure descriptions at this site, some in both English and Spanish.

Glossary

accreditation: the process of ensuring that all equipment, supplies, and procedures of an inspected facility meet or surpass the high expectations of one of two agencies—the American Association of Accredited Ambulatory Surgical Facilities (AAAASF) and the Accreditation Association for Ambulatory Health Care (AAAHC). These agencies inspect surgical centers and make sure they meet the highest standards of safety for patients.

Accreditation Association for Ambulatory Health Care (AAAHC): one of two agencies responsible for inspecting surgical centers and making sure that they meet the highest standards of safety for patients. To be accredited by the AAAHC, a facility's equipment, supplies, and procedures must meet or surpass extremely high expectations.

American Association of Accredited Ambulatory Surgical Facilities (AAAASF): one of two agencies responsible for inspecting surgical centers and ensuring that they meet the highest standards of safety for patients. To be accredited by the AAAASF, a facility's equipment, supplies, and procedures must meet or surpass extremely high expectations.

American Board of Medical Specialties (ABMS): the overall encompassing body of the medical world and the only entity that lists all of the various medical boards. The ABMS consists of 24 approved medical specialty boards, one of which is the American Board of Plastic Surgery (ABPS). Certification by the ABMS indicates that surgeons are performing to the highest standard of their profession.

American Board of Plastic Surgery (ABPS): a board within the American Board of Medical Specialties that focuses specifically on plastic surgery.

American Society of Plastic Surgeons (ASPS): the largest agency that focuses specifically on plastic surgery in the world, the ASPS helps prospective patients find board-certified plastic surgeons in their area.

anchor technique: a breast reduction method that leaves an anchor-shaped scar. The anchor method is considered an inferior-pedicle technique.

anesthesiologist: physician trained to administer anesthesia.

antibiotic: medication created from mold or bacterium that wards off infection.

antimicrobial soap: cleanser that prevents infection. Surgeons often recommend that patients wash with antimicrobial soap before undergoing surgery.

areola of the breast: pigmented area surrounding the nipple.

augmentation: process of enlargement, often referring to breast surgery.

baseline mammogram: a mammogram that will show what a patient's "normal" is to enable future mammograms to display any changes that could be troublesome. Women over forty often are advised to acquire a baseline mammogram before undergoing surgery.

betadine: an antiseptic solution painted on the chest with a scrub brush to sterilize the entire area in which a surgical procedure will be performed.

blood chemistry test: a procedure that screens for problems with levels of potassium, sodium, creatinine, fasting glucose, total cholesterol and HDL cholesterol.

blood pregnancy test: procedure during which blood is drawn in order to determine whether a pregnancy exists. Often, surgeons request a blood pregnancy test at the consultation.

bra strap grooving: deep dips in shoulders caused by bra straps being pulled down by large, pendulous breasts. This symptom is a common complaint of many women exploring breast reduction surgery.

breast bud: breasts forming small peaks as nipples swell and tenderness sets in during early breast development.

breast ducts: tube-shaped structures that carry breast milk.

breast examination: a painless procedure performed by a medical professional that consists of a visual assessment followed by a breast, armpit, and collarbone area exam to ensure that no lumps that could be cancerous are present.

breast implant: a sac filled with fluid or gel that is inserted either under breast tissue or under the chest wall to enhance the breast. Breast implants are usually filled with silicone or saline.

breast lift (mastopexy): a breast surgery procedure during which excess skin, fat, and tissue are removed in order to raise sagging breasts to a desired level. Less than 500 grams of fat and breast tissue is removed from each breast in order for a procedure to be considered a breast lift and not a breast reduction.

breast lift with augmentation: a breast surgery procedure during which excess skin, fat, and tissue are removed and an implant is inserted in order to raise sagging breasts to desired level and enhance their size, fullness, and firmness.

breast lobules: small lobes in the breast containing breast milk.

breast reduction: a breast surgery procedure during which at least 500 grams of breast tissue and fat are removed. Contrary to popular belief, breast reduction does not usually include liposuction; instead, fat, breast tissue, and extra skin are removed surgically. Two common breast reduction methods are the lollipop technique and the anchor technique.

capsular contracture: a complication which occurs when the scar or the capsule surrounding the implant begins to tighten, thus causing the breast to feel hard. Capsular contracture is rectified either by removing the implant or operating on the breast's scar tissue.

certification: a process by which a select group of surgeons is approved by the American Board of Medical Specialties. Certification by this agency means that surgeons are performing to the highest standard of their profession.

chest X-ray: a procedure which screens for lung masses or abnormalities.

complete blood count (CBC): a screening and diagnostic test for a variety of diseases. It indicates problems with fluid volume, loss of blood, abnormal blood cells, infection, allergies, and clotting.

compression stockings: plastic surgical device wrapped around patients' legs to improve circulation to lower extremities while under anesthesia. The compression stockings inflate and deflate throughout surgery to keep blood flowing.

CT (computed tomography) scan: a screening procedure using X-rays to view organs and other body structures. Also called a CAT (computerized axial tomography) scan.

consultation: the initial meeting with a potential surgeon during which a patient learns about the surgical process; whether he or she is a candidate for surgery, and risks, probable outcomes, and cost of surgery. This is the time when patients also make sure they feel a rapport with the surgeon.

drainage tubes: small, plastic tubes about three millimeters in diameter that are inserted into surgical incisions during breast reduction surgery to greatly diminish risk of hematoma and seratoma.

drains: spherical containers at the end of drainage tubes that catch excess fluid.

ECG (electrocardiogram): a painless screening procedure that records the electrical activity of the heart and screens for heart disease. Electrodes are affixed to the chest, arms and legs. It may also include a stress test where patients may be expected to perform some sort of physical activity.

estrogen: a hormone produced by the ovaries, placenta, testes, and adrenal cortex that controls growth, maturation, and the menstrual cycle.

general anesthesia: method used to stop pain from being felt during a procedure or surgery.

general practitioner: physician trained to care for all basic medical conditions.

genes: space on chromosomes dedicated to heredity and containing DNA.

gynecologist: physician specializing in female genitalia, endocrinology, and reproduction.

hematoma: a pooling of blood under the skin.

hypertrophic scar: overdeveloped scars that may be thick, red, and ropy.

incision: a cut made through the skin with a knife or laser during a surgical procedure.

inferior-based pedicle technique: procedure during which skin from the lower portion of the breast remains connected to the nipple and areola.

intravenous: inside a vein.

IV: *see intravenous*

keloid: a raised, thick, irregular scar caused by excessive tissue growth at the site of an incision or wound.

liposuction: process of removing undesirable fat with suction tubes.

local anesthesia: method used to block pain sensations in a region of the body.

lollipop technique: the breast reduction method that uses vertical incisions, resulting in a scar that resembles a lollipop.

mammogram: a low-powered X-ray method that displays the entire inner structure of the breast. It's used to screen for a variety of breast maladies, the most common of which is cancer.

mammoplasty: a generic term for cosmetic surgery for the breasts

mastopexy: breast lift

medical team: a group of several professionals, including an anesthesiologist, a surgeon, a physician technician, and two or three nurses, who participate in the surgical process.

MRI (magnetic resonance imaging): diagnostic procedure using magnetic fields and radio waves to view organs and other body structures.

pectoral muscles: chest wall, under which breast implants are often placed.

physical examination: a physician's assessment of a patient's vital signs: height, weight, blood pressure, pulse, temperature, and so forth. Blood is drawn to screen for disease and organ malfunction. The physician will also listen for lung functioning and heartbeat. During a breast consultation, a plastic surgeon will conduct a more specific physical examination that includes evaluation of shoulder bra strap grooving, current nipple sensitivity, nipple position, distance between different parts of the breast, breast size, breast symmetry, chest wall size, and breast shape.

plastic surgeon: a medical doctor who specializes in reducing scarring and disfigurement from accidents, birth defects, and diseases. A cosmetic plastic surgeon specializes in aesthetic improvement of the face and body via surgery.

ptosis: sagging.

radiologist: physician trained to therapeutically interpret X-rays.

reduction mammaplasty: surgery to reduce size and weight of breasts.

saline: mixture of salt and water often used in breast implants.

seroma: a pooling of fluid under the skin.

silicone: a synthetic polymer often used in

breast implants in the past. Silicone implants are awaiting the FDA's final approval, but can be used only in special cases until its proven that they are not dangerous.

Steri-Strips: pieces of surgical tape designed to hold together and protect sutured incisions. Steri-strips provide an external alternative to traditional stitches, fall off on their own, and do not cause any pain. They are commonly known as "butterfly stitches."

superior-based pedicle technique: procedure during which skin from the upper portion of the breast stays connected to the nipple and areola during surgery.

support garment: bra designed to restrict movement after surgery until breasts have begun to heal.

surgical dressing: bandages wrapped around operation area of body by surgeon to absorb excess fluid and keep incisions protected. After breast surgery, the surgical dressing is covered by a surgical support garment.

surgical center: a facility used by a surgeon to perform surgical procedures. Surgical centers may or may not be accredited by the American Association of Accredited Ambulatory Surgical Facilities (AAAASF) or the Accreditation Association for Ambulatory Health Care (AAAHC).

sutures: surgical stitches.

urine pregnancy test: a procedure during which urine is evaluated in order to determine whether a pregnancy exists. Often, a surgeon will request a urine pregnancy test the day of surgery.

vertical technique: the breast reduction method that uses vertical incisions, resulting in a scar that resembles a lollipop. Also called the lollipop technique.

virginal breast hypertrophy: the condition of having developed large breasts at a very early age, usually during grade school.

Index

A

abnormal blood cells, 34
accreditation, 19
Accreditation Association for Ambulatory Health Care (AAAHC), 19
addiction, 75
alcohol consumption, 10, 36, 79
allergies, 34
allergic reaction to anesthesia, 52
American Association of Accredited Ambulatory Surgical Facilities (AAAASF), 19
American Board of Plastic Surgery, 17
American Board of Surgery, 17
American Society of Plastic Surgeons (ASPS), 7, 15, 52, 53, 55
anchor incision, 45, 46, 68
    scars, 46
anemia, 33, 34
    symptoms, 33, 34
anesthesia, 42, 44, 79
    allergic reaction, 52
anesthesiologist, 43
antibiotic, 75
antimicrobial soap, 38

areola, 5, 46, 47
    reduction, 48
aspiration pneumonia, 37
aspirin, 35
asymmetry, 48, 53
augmentation, 62–71

B

back pain, 8
bank loan options, 29
bathing, 38
before and after photographs, 26, 27
blood cells, 44
blood chemistry test, 34
blood clots, 44
blood gases, 44
blood pregnancy test, 33
blood thinners, 35, 36
board certification, 16, 17
body mass index (BMI), 28
bra, 77
bra size, 25
bra strap grooving, 8, 25
breast
    anatomy, 5, 6
    growth, 5, 6, 9
    massage, 53, 79

    maturation, 6
    measurements, 25
    milk, 57
    rashes, 8
    tenderness, 55
breast augmentation, 62–71
breast bud, 5
breast cancer, 25, 33, 69
breast development, 5, 6, 9
    stages, 5
breast duct, 6
breast examination, 25
breast fat, 6
breast implants, 63–71
    breastfeeding, 68
    candidates for, 68
    complications, 67
    disadvantages, 67, 68
    placement, 66–68
    pregnancy, 68
    shapes, 65
    sizes, 66
    subglandular placement, 67–69
    submuscular placement, 66, 67, 69
    textures, 65
    types, 63–65

breast lift with augmentation, 63–71
    complications, 69
    risk factors, 69
breast lifts, 7, 60–71
    candidates for, 62
breast reduction surgery
    candidates for, 8, 9
    complications, 26, 52–55
    cost, 27, 28
    definition, 7
    incision techniques, 45–47
    preparation for, 32–39
    procedure, 42–57
    reasons for, 8
    recovery, 50, 51
    risk factors, 52–55
    risks, 26
    side effects, 47, 50, 51
breast symmetry, 25, 43, 47
breastfeeding, 6, 9, 56, 57, 61
    effect of anesthesia, 9
breathing tube, 45
bruising, 50, 55, 74, 76

C

calcium deposits, 69
candidates for

breast lifts, 62
breast reduction surgery, 8, 9
implants, 68
capsular contracture, 67–69
caregiver, 36
causes of sagging breasts, 61
chest X-ray, 34
choosing a plastic surgeon, 14–19
    referrals, 15
circumareolar incision, 62
clotting ability, 34
complete blood count (CBC), 33, 34
complications
    breast reduction surgery, 52–55
compression stockings, 44
consultation, 22–29
contraceptives, 7
cost, 27, 28, 71

D

death of skin,
    see necrosis
deep vein thrombosis (DVT), 44
depression, 51
diabetes, 8, 32
draining tubes, 48, 49, 75, 76

removal, 77, 79
driving, 78
droopy breasts, 60
    see also ptosis

E

electrocardiogram (EKG) or (ECG), 34
estrogen, 6
replacement therapy, 7
exercise, 10, 78

F

fat necrosis, 53, 54
fees, 27, 28, 71
follow-up care, 74–79
food intake, 38

G

general anesthesia, 44
general practitioner, 10, 15
genetics, 6
gynecologist, 15

H

hardening of breast tissue, 55
    see also capsular contracture
health history, 8

hemoglobin, 44

hematoma, 48, 54

   draining, 54

hormones, 5, 6

hospital, 19, 42

hypertrophic scar, 55, 79

I

implants, 63–71

   affect on mammogram, 69, 70

   breastfeeding, 68

   candidates for, 68

   complications, 67

   disadvantages, 67, 68

   fees, 71

   placement, 66–68

   pregnancy, 68

   saline, 64, 69

   shapes, 65

   shifting, 69

   silicone, 64, 65

   sizes, 66

   subglandular placement, 67–69

   submuscular placement, 66–69

   textures, 65

   types, 63–65

incision techniques, 45–47

infection, 34, 52, 75

inferior-based pedicle technique, 46

inflammatory phase of healing, 56

informed consent form, 29

inframammary fold, 46, 60

insurance, 9, 27, 28

   criteria, 28

intermittent sequential compression devices (SCD's), 44

Internet, 15

intravenous (IV) line, 42

K

keloid scar, 10, 11, 46, 55, 79

L

lab tests, 32–34

lactation, 6

licensing criteria, 17

liposuction, 57, 79

lobules, 5

lollipop incision, 45–47, 62, 68

loss of blood, 34

lymph nodes, 25

M

magnetic resonance imaging (MRI), 70

mammogram, 33, 67

marijuana, 10

mastitis, 25

mastopexy

   see breast lift

medical clearance, 32

medical history, 8, 25, 32

medical records, 22

medical team, 43

medications to avoid, 35, 36

menopause, 7, 61

menstruation, 5

metabolic phase of healing, 56

milk duct, 5

N

nail polish, 38

nausea, 37

neck pain, 8

necrosis, 53, 54

nicotine, 10, 34

   gum, 35

   lozenges, 35

patches, 35
nipple, 5, 46, 47, 60
    discharge, 25
    position, 25
    sensitivity, 25, 52
numbness, 50
nutrition plan, 10

O

obesity, 9
oral contraceptives, 7
ovary production, 5

P

pain management, 74, 75, 79
pain medication, 75
pathology report, 27
patient references, 27
pectoralis major muscle, 5, 66, 67
permanent breast size, 6
physical examination, 32–34
physical symptoms, 28
physician technician, 43
pigment changes, 53
pituitary gland, 5
plastic surgeon
    choosing, 14–19

consultation, 22–29
experience, 17
procedure, 42–57
qualifications, 15–19
training, 15–19
post-menopause estrogen replacement, 7
post-surgery care, 50, 51
posture, 8
pre-operative medical clearance, 32
pre-operative photographs, 26, 27
pre-operative procedures, 37
pregnancy, 6, 9, 61, 62
pregnancy test
    types, 33
preparation for breast reduction surgery, 32–39
previous surgeries, 22
pseudoptosis, 60
ptosis of breasts, 60–62
    degrees, 60, 61
puberty, 5–6, 8
pulse oximeter, 44

R

radiologist, 33, 69, 70

recertification, 17
reconstructive surgery, 28
recovery, 50, 51
recovery at home, 37, 78
recovery room, 43
red blood cells, 33
reduction mammoplasty, 7
    see also breast reduction surgery
referrals, 15
remodeling phase of healing, 56
residency, 16
returning to work, 78, 79
revisional surgery, 79
ripples in skin, 68
risk factors
    breast reduction surgery, 52–55
    breast implants, 67

S

saline implants, 64, 69
scars, 10, 11, 51, 55, 79
second consultations, 23
self-confidence, 82–85
self-pay options, 29
seroma, 48, 54
serum, 48

sexual activity, 8, 79

shoulder pain, 8

side effects
    of breast reduction surgery, 47
    breast reduction surgery, 50, 51

silicone implants, 64, 65

smoking, 10, 79
    cessation aids, 35
    quitting, 34, 35

soreness, 50

sports activity, 8

stages of healing, 56

state medical board, 18

Steri-strips, 49, 77

steroid use, 10

stress test, 34

subglandular implant placement, 67, 68

submuscular implant placement, 66, 67

sun exposure, 78

superior-based pedicle technique, 47

supero-medial-based pedicle technique, 47

supplements, 35

support garment, 50, 74, 76, 77

surgical center, 19, 42, 43, 79

surgical dressing, 76, 77

surgical markings, 43

surgical support bra, 77

suture, 47, 49, 77
    absorbable, 77

swelling, 50, 55, 74, 76

symmetry, 25, 43, 47

T

thyroid disorders, 32

U

undermining, 49

urine pregnancy test, 33

V

vertical technique
    see lollipop incision

virginal breast hypertrophy, 9

W

weight gain, 7, 61

weight loss program, 10

X

X-ray, 33–34, 69

About the Authors

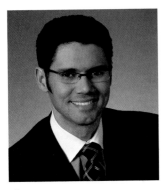

"My approach to cosmetic breast surgery is to fully understand the nature of each patient's concerns about her breasts both physically and emotionally. With this awareness I can then tailor each procedure to fully achieve the patients goals."

Alain Polynice, M.D.

Alain Polynice, MD is a plastic surgeon in private practice with The Plastic Surgery Associates of New York, with offices in New York City and Westchester, New York. He performs cosmetic surgery at a variety of private surgery centers and hospitals in the New York metropolitan area. Dr. Polynice is board certified by the American Board of Plastic Surgery. Upon completing his residency in plastic and reconstructive surgery at the world-renowned Mayo Clinic in Rochester, Minnesota, Dr. Polynice completed a six-month traveling fellowship throughout the United States, Australia, Asia, and Europe.

Dr. Polynice has worked with leaders in the fields of body and facial plastic surgery. He has cutting edge experience in facial rejuvenation, body contouring, and breast reconstruction. His international background and training also give him keen insight into the needs of patients across many cultural lines. Dr. Polynice is fluent in the French and Spanish languages.

Dr. Polynice has been published in several peer reviewed medical journals. He is a member of the New York Regional Society of Plastic Surgery, the American Society of Plastic Surgery, and the American Burn Association. Dr. Polynice has an academic appointment at New York Medical College as assistant clinical professor of surgery; there he is closely involved in teaching and molding young plastic surgeons in training. Dr. Polynice may be reached through his Web site: **www.plasticsurgeryassociatesny.com.**

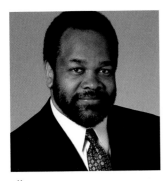

"My goal is to help improve a patient's quality of life. Thanks to major advances in recent years, we have dramatically improved our ability to surgically restore or create a more pleasing and appealing balance in one's appearance."

Aloysius G. Smith, M.D.

Aloysius G. Smith, MD is a plastic surgeon in private practice with the Plastic Surgery Associates of New York in New York City and Yonkers, New York. He is board certified by the American Board of Plastic Surgery and the American Board of Surgery. Dr. Smith received his fellowship training in plastic and reconstructive surgery at the world-renowned Mayo Clinic, Rochester, Minnesota. Dr. Smith has been a specialist in reconstructive and plastic surgery for twenty years practicing in Manhattan, Yonkers, and the Bronx, NY.

Dr. Smith is director of plastic surgery at St. Joseph's Hospital and Medical Center, Our Lady of Mercy Medical Center and Lincoln Medical, and Mental Health Center in New York. His academic appointments include assistant professor of surgery at New York Medical College, where he is involved in training the next generation of plastic surgeons in the latest surgical knowledge and techniques. Dr. Smith may be reached through his Web site: **www.plasticsurgeryassociatesny.com.**